RHEUMATOID ARTHRITIS UNMASKED:
10 DANGERS
OF
RHEUMATOID DISEASE

Kelly O'Neill Young

Printed in the United States of America
First Edition
ISBN-13: 978-0-9989374-7-2

Cover Illustration Copyright © 2017 by Mary Khristyne New

RA Patient Insights, LLC
Orlando, Florida

RAwarrior.com/rheumatoidarthritisunmasked

DEDICATION

This book is dedicated to my grandfather,
Samuel Monroe Phillips,
who fought rheumatoid disease
the same way almost every person does: privately.

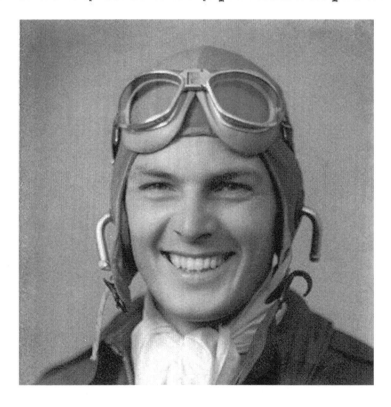

ACKNOWLEDGEMENTS

First, I would like to acknowledge my Mom, Judy, who has been my biggest fan. Her faith in me can lift me up over any challenge.

I wrote this book for my five extraordinary children, the lights of my life. They have brought me all of the joy a mother could ask for.

My daughter Katie Beth, the talented scientist who has been my "partner in crime" from day one. We stood together, held on tight, and propelled each other forward to try to change the world.

My daughter Mary Khris, the talented artist who designed my spear-pen logo, setting me on a path to eventually need the crumbling mask she created for the cover to this book.

The words of reader named Jay Wood put things in motion that led me here. It's all his fault.

The readers of my blog, who not only turn to me for help, but also freely help me and one another in return, are the sweetest and strongest community a person could find.

My dear Leslie for admiring me no matter what I can't do, but never forgetting what I did before rheumatoid disease.

Friends who have believed in me enough to inspire me to keep going until this was finished: Dave deBronkart, John Davis, Dana Symons, Alex Bangs, John Holt, Vi Dagdigian, and Bob West.

My oldest friend Julie Holdren Lydell who was good enough to teach me HTML over the phone one day. A true story about the birth of RA Warrior.

The whole board of the Rheumatoid Patient Foundation, past, present, and future, for sharing the dream of making life better for people with RD.

Dr. R. Franklin Adams, Rheumatic Disease specialist, for speaking the truth of what's behind the mask.

Barb and Paul who have been so steadfast in helping our family through the hardest time.

FOREWORD

Since I first had lunch with Kelly Young at the American College of Rheumatology annual scientific meeting several years ago, I have known that she truly is *RA Warrior*. In her fight to better the lives of patients, I have heard her give powerful presentations to my fellow physicians and watched her lead a team to produce innovative research. Kelly has accomplished these things while living with rheumatoid disease (RD) herself. As a matter of fact, her struggles with getting a diagnosis and finding effective treatment highlight major challenges in rheumatology.

Kelly is not only a patient journalist and an effective advocate for patients, but through her online community, she is also counselor to many thousands of people living with rheumatoid disease (RD). This has equipped her with vast knowledge and experience to understand the disease. *Rheumatoid Arthritis Unmasked* follows the gradual recognition of various aspects of this disease through clinical research, relying on hundreds of academic studies. Kelly takes the reader on a tour de force through that history of RD, demonstrating her impressive knowledge of the scientific literature in this work.

As a person, Kelly is delightful, intelligent, warm, and very funny. As the reader will soon discover, Kelly gives a strong voice to all people living with rheumatoid disease (PRD). She fearlessly raises awareness of the many gaps in the general understanding of this disease. As I read the book, I was mindful that this includes patient-physician communication, and perhaps most importantly, empathy toward those suffering the ravages of this disease.

Kelly argues persuasively that the current name of the disease, rheumatoid arthritis, is a major problem. She explains how the disease that patients experience is inconsistent with the way the disease is defined, which contributes to widespread misunderstanding of the disease. She passionately describes how basic misconceptions of this disease, among both the medical and lay communities, contribute to adverse health outcomes for PRD.

Although the symptom of arthritis is a dominant manifestation of the disease, the label of "arthritis" misleads physicians to narrowly focus on the articular manifestations in their clinical assessments. Rheumatologists focus on identifying swollen joints as the key defining manifestation of the disease, when in truth, there are many diverse manifestations that vary greatly between patients and in the same patient over time. The disease deserves a new name that should ultimately not only recognize the scientific understanding of the disease but also identify its nature as a serious systemic autoimmune inflammatory disease.

On many levels, we need the greater awareness of the true nature of RD that *Rheumatoid Arthritis Unmasked* brings. First, we need health care professionals to become more aware of RD's systemic manifestations and of the inherent limitations of current diagnostic assessments and disease-modifying treatments. Second, we need awareness of the unmet needs for patients living with rheumatic diseases by those individuals who make decisions about research funding. Third, we need greater awareness in the broader population about the plight of people living with rheumatoid disease.

In considering these necessary changes, it is important for all to imagine what it would be like to live a life filled with joint pain, profound fatigue and exertion intolerance, loss of physical function, and even feeling a loss of self. Contemplating this would promote appropriate empathy toward PRD.

With this book, Kelly Young makes an important contribution to the patient revolution. She advances the cause of the Rheumatoid Patient Foundation and patient advocacy overall. Her effective advocacy will bring increased participation of patients in their health care decisions, and hopefully, improved treatment options for all of the various manifestations of this disease. In this text, she has successfully "unmasked" RD, demonstrating the true nature of this morbid and mortal disease to all.

John M. Davis III, M.D.
Practice Chair, Division of Rheumatology, Department of Internal Medicine
Mayo Clinic
Rochester, MN

TABLE OF CONTENTS

Author's Note

It was my son's first birthday—the day I was finally diagnosed with RA. I'll always remember it. Months of researching to figure out what was wrong and years of doctors assuring me "No, you couldn't have RA" were over in one terrible confusing moment. If my life were a play, that would be the turning point where everything began to move in a different direction. Most of the things I'd loved doing were instantly out of reach. Decades of exhaustive efforts to be strong and healthy went up in smoke. Friendships I'd counted on went down in flames.

Before that time, I had been a hardworking self-reliant proud daughter of a Marine. Whether it was homeschooling, ministry, or DIY projects, I always gave my best effort and left it all on the field. I'm pretty sure my kids thought I was invincible. Then I got sick. In some ways, that was when their childhood ended. The Momma who did everything for them was gone. Instead, they had to help me. They took over many chores, helped me take care of the baby, and even washed my hair because I couldn't raise my arms.

The physical struggles were made worse by the way friends and family, neighbors and church folks reacted. They all seemed to be sure that I was not really sick, but even if I were, they knew just the cure—Tylenol, juice, magnetic bracelets, and confessing my hidden sins. No one adjusted their expectations of me or offered to help. Instead they sat me down to straighten me out.

It seemed like every day there was a new symptom in a joint I'd never heard of before. And pain. Up until then, the worst pain I'd ever experienced had been the natural home births of my five children. Now, I lived with pain on that scale every day. I was so alone and confused.

I started listening to anyone I could find with the disease. When I heard someone's cousin or sister had RA, I asked them to call me. For hours every day, I read everything about the disease I could get—at the library and online. The discrepancies between the descriptions of the disease and what patients actually lived with amazed me. How could something this common be so misunderstood?

Patients' stories tugged at my heart. They'd suffered the same things I had—earth-shattering pain, instant disability, and an endless stream of weird symptoms, like a jaw stuck shut, mysterious black circles at the toenail cuticle, and losing my voice for weeks at a time. Who knew that a disease this far-reaching and peculiar even existed?

Except for my kids and my best friend, everywhere I turned people seemed to think I was crazy. Everywhere except for one place—the community of patients I began to gather online. In our RA Warrior community, we helped each other find ways to still be ourselves despite what the disease had stolen. I told people what I wished someone had told me. I told them, "You're not crazy. It's a crazy disease." For several years, I worked hard to help people with RA by bringing them accurate information and bringing their stories back to government, the pharmaceutical industry and the medical community. And I received so much joy and friendship from people in return.

My name, Kelly, is a Gaelic word meaning "warrior." That meaning took on new significance now. My Quest was to help people with RA fight back in every way possible. But giving speeches, writing hundreds of articles, or making videos wasn't enough. Patients need and deserve more. They need someone to tell the whole truth about the disease. Strangely, the truth is the opposite of what is commonly believed: *The disease is not less than what it seems. It's much more.*

I could see it plainly: rheumatoid arthritis is actually rheumatoid disease (RD). My grandfather was not the only victim of the RD mortality gap[1] that I knew. I have talked with thousands of people about their symptoms and their struggles. One by one, I've told them: "I believe you. Yes this can be caused by RD. Now, go see a specialist doctor and take good care of yourself." This is my reason for writing this book: with it, I can tell thousands more.

But a book couldn't just be a list of things to watch out for, a list of things I've learned in my years as an advocate. To be reliable, it had to be fully documented. It had to be something doctors could read too, and know it's valid. And so, to be sure, I did not rely on my own experience as a patient, journalist, or advocate. I have used hundreds of research articles and peer reviewed studies in writing this book.

I began this book in 2013, but it has taken me a long time to finish it. In recent years, my RD has advanced and the work has slowed. The book seemed to become my Impossible Dream. In 2017, I was stirred with a sense of urgency. Several events in my family and with my own RD made me realize I must finish this book—and the next one that is partly written—as soon as possible. It is difficult since my joints don't allow me to type normally any more and my eyes are sore. But I know I must put these facts into the hands of people with RD so they can fight back against this malevolent disease. I plan to put this book into the hands of as many clinicians as possible so that they will be better equipped to help right the unrightable wrong of RD.

Kelly O'Neill Young
RA Warrior
July 31, 2017
Orlando, Florida

---

[1] A mortality gap is excess mortality in any particular group including people of a certain gender, race, or geographic region.

INTRODUCTION

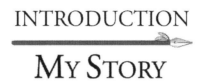

MY STORY

How I recognized the confusion about the nature of the disease

Why does RA need to be unmasked?

What is rheumatoid arthritis (RA) really? Does it make any difference how we understand it? Why do patients and doctors need to be warned about the *10 Dangers of Rheumatoid Disease*?

Unfortunately, the general medical perception of RA is wholly inadequate. Most patients are also sadly unaware of serious health dangers related to RA, and it's difficult for them to find accurate information. When they are diagnosed with "arthritis," the last thing they expect is a disease that affects their heart or their lungs.

But that is what rheumatoid disease (RD) does.

For people who live with it, being uninformed that RA is actually RD can have obvious consequences. They might see their problems as having separate causes. Imagine that a person is a little short of breath, but also unable to use her hands or even walk. Which one seems more urgent? If you can't stand up, put on a shirt, or hold a fork, you will seek medical attention for your joints. And too often being short of breath—or fatigued—will take a back seat to being able to function. However, as you will read, being short of breath could be a serious sign of other problems caused by the disease.

What difference will it make if we unmask RA?

This book will answer that question with evidence from medical research. But it will do more than that. Since I am a patient who works with other patients, I also see the disease from the vantage point of the patient experience. Here's a glimpse into my own story.

Evolving joints, rashes, and fears

When I was thirteen years old, I awoke with my hands in fists. One at a time, I pried each finger straight. I didn't give it much thought, but the stiff fingers and the prying process was repeated every morning for a few weeks. And then the stiffness stopped. That experience was my initiation into two aspects of RA that would characterize much of my future life: *enduring pain* and *accepting baffling symptoms.*

Twenty-six years later, I was diagnosed with full-blown RA. Although the intervening years had included many periodic symmetrical flares of feet, hips, and shoulders, no one was more shocked than I was to finally learn I had RA. Normal ESR (erythrocyte sedimentation rate) tests had assured uninformed doctors—and ignorant me—that it was impossible I had RA.

Nevertheless, during the year after diagnosis, the disease spread through my body like two long identical rows of dominoes, symmetrically inflaming every joint and acquainting me with some I hadn't known existed. My feet joints were the first to become unusable and swell conspicuously. I was concerned since there was no explanation for this intense inflammation of metatarsophalangeal (MTP) joints on both feet. I had merely bumped one toe joint on a metal stool leg, and the inflammation spread to other toe joints. It was almost impossible to walk, like standing on sharp rocks beneath the skin.

Next came sudden pain in both shoulders that could only be compared to pain during childbirth without any medication. One night at 2 a.m., I awoke with a shoulder hurting so badly, it felt like I'd been shot. I struggled to get up and take four Advil, but that medicine did nothing for the pain. At 3 a.m.—exactly an hour later—the other shoulder started hurting the same way. After a couple hours of agony, I wanted to go to the emergency room, but my husband didn't agree. At this point, I suspected some kind of systemic illness, but he was right: I had no evidence. The next week, my knees joined the chorus of pain.

To cope, I relied heavily on my years of experience of ignoring painful symptoms. However, this became impossible because oftentimes I could not move my arms (shoulders) or walk (feet or knees). Through childbirth and spine injuries, I had learned to endure severe pain quietly by breathing deeply and focusing on other things. But there were many times I couldn't force my frozen or weak joints to move, and determination wasn't enough to help that. It wasn't just pain—there was stiffness and weakness I could not always overcome.

During the first few weeks, the primary care physician dismissed my symptoms, looked past me, and explicitly assured my husband that I was "perfectly healthy" because "there is no illness that does this."

Meanwhile, watching my symptoms evolve, the podiatrist who treated my feet suspected RA. That practice provided me over a decade of good care, mainly because the doctors have always offered me proper medical care instead of dismissing my symptoms. God bless Dr. David Campbell and Dr. Mark Beylin.

Too many strange symptoms to call it arthritis

Along with joint symptoms came daily fevers and bright red symmetrical rashes covering both arms. I tried to ignore those too, since few people in my life acknowledged that there was any problem. Some of my friends and family, and even people at church insisted nothing was wrong with me. Every day there were new tactless remarks or endless recommendations to cure my suspiciously sudden disability. They offered Tylenol arthritis, açai juice, magic magnets, copper jewelry, and changing my sinful heart. When people refused to adjust their expectations of what I could do, I wondered how unlucky I could be, surrounded by unsympathetic people who refused to help. However, since then, hundreds of people with rheumatoid disease have shared similarly vexing stories. I learned that, for many, dealing with inappropriate responses from others is part of the RD experience.

During those early months, the skin on my face and neck would suddenly turn hot red every day. This was not blushing; it was redder than blushing. I had never blushed before, since I have a tanned olive complexion. But, since no one understood what was wrong, that symptom was ignored like everything else.

Honestly, the symptoms were something more than confusing to me: they were frightening. Since everyone dismissed my strange symptoms, I learned to stay quiet. But this did not stop the disease from progressing.

I now know that some of my symptoms, including the black circles on my toes, could be explained by rheumatoid vasculitis,[1] a "complication" of rheumatoid disease with which I was later diagnosed. Perhaps the red face was related to that.

This is only a glimpse of my story, but it still feels strange and awkward to share. No one wants to admit to crazy-sounding symptoms. Even now that I've heard many surprising stories from other patients, I'm uncomfortable writing this because what happened to me sounds so peculiar.

I can't explain it all. But I am certain of this: *Arthritis is not the right word to describe what was happening to me.*

Was there no one else like me?

Finally diagnosed, I was treated with the maximum (25mg injectable) dose of methotrexate and a biologic. I quickly adjusted my life to accommodate regular medications, putting considerable trust in my new rheumatologist and her recommendations. I put all of my effort into getting well. I bought pill organizers for medicines and supplements. I gave myself weekly shots. So as not to appear too sick in front of the kids, I would secretly inject myself in the hotel bathroom on family trips. And I won several inevitable arguments with our insurance company. I stoically endured hair loss, episodes of severe nausea, and repeated skin infections. With my immune system suppressed,[2] I was treated first for pneumonia and then a kidney infection. Other infections included a six-month long UTI and cellulitis. Eventually, side effects would include six months of severe bronchitis from one biologic medication and sudden onset of a swollen liver with another. Yet I was fully compliant, never missing doses or fussing about side effects, even with a doubled-dose of a TNF-a inhibitor for over a year.

However, new dominoes continued to fall. I repeatedly asked my doctor, "When will I be able to run again?" She often told me, "Most people get better" and I enthusiastically believed it was just a matter of time. Eventually, the rheumatologist admitted defeat, saying that I had "become atypical" by not responding well to medication. The one biologic I'd used for three years was the only one which that practice prescribed at the time.

I didn't know anyone else with RA and did not know where to turn. Still strongly determined to get my life back, I spent substantial time researching online. I simply wanted to find answers when the doctor admitted not knowing what to do next. Online, I learned more about other biologic medicines—*and other patients.*

It didn't take long to see that I was not alone. And it became obvious that I was not atypical. *Most people with RA have had systemic symptoms, varying indicators, and inadequate responses to treatments.* It's also extremely common for RA patients to be told they are "atypical." The more I read, the more surprised I was to grasp a peculiar fact: The disease experienced by patients was not reliably reflected in most medical literature.[3]

The discrepancies I saw led me to create the resource called *rawarrior.com* in 2009, which now contains about 900 articles related to RA and its treatment. Meanwhile, I wrote for other publications, gave public speeches to create awareness of RA, and became involved in research. After working full-time with patients and reading research, I realized the need for an organization to represent the interests of patients, as exists for most other health conditions. Together with several other patients, I founded the Rheumatoid Patient Foundation (RPF) in 2011.[4]

Patients hate the "a" word.

By late 2008, there were already forum discussions and blogs that advocated changing the name of RA. As I read comments by patients, I was not convinced that changing the name was achievable or essential. Would a new name affect patients' treatments? Would it improve RA awareness? Yes it might, but I thought we could likely accomplish these efforts without a name change. Would the establishment listen to patients' objections about the name seeing as it already discounted our descriptions of the disease? I doubted it.

Yet, most people who live with this systemic disease quickly grow to hate the way it is politely dismissed as "a type of arthritis," creating confusion and needless added problems. When people with rheumatoid disease (PRD) mention their diagnosis as "RA," others insist that their "arthritis" is the same. Within weeks of diagnosis, most PRD learn it's nearly impossible to convince others—even doctors—of the systemic nature of their illness or the wide-ranging extent of their medical problems. Patients often determine that it is too difficult a struggle to explain or defend the disease in either personal or medical settings.

One thing links virtually every story or discussion about misperceptions related to RA: the word *arthritis*.

I've read hundreds of patient descriptions of how they invent alternate ways to describe their diagnosis such as a "lupus-like condition" or an "immune system disease." Patients avoid the use of the "a" word because as soon as it is uttered, a wrong opinion is formed about the nature of their diagnosis.

Having the unique vantage point of hearing from tens of thousands of RA patients personally and living with the disease myself, I had been converted. It is unmistakable: rheumatoid arthritis is actually rheumatoid disease.

I became convinced the language must be changed in order to

bring more complete treatment and better outcomes for patients. And I began to spearhead a movement to accomplish that. The Rheumatoid Patient Foundation does not have the "a" word in its name because we are looking forward to the time when people with rheumatoid disease will be treated according to distinct disease mechanisms and live longer healthier lives as their systemic disease is alleviated.

In my Granddad's heart, rheumatoid arthritis was a disease

Rheumatoid is a disease whether we acknowledge it or not. With or without our acknowledgement, the disease makes patients ill as it attacks various systems in their bodies. If we pretend that rheumatoid is simply "a type of arthritis," eyes will still be sore, lungs will still be damaged, and people like my Granddad will still die from its cumulative effects. To a patient's body, RA is a disease, whatever others may call it.

Will a name change make any difference? If we acknowledge RA as a disease, calling it "rheumatoid disease," what will be gained by updating the label? Who will benefit? What historical precedent is there for such a change? *This book will show you why the change is necessary for patients and for the medical community to better fight this dangerous disease.*

Another generation should not suffer.

This book is dedicated to my Granddad, Monroe Phillips, who fought rheumatoid disease the same way almost every patient does: privately.[5, 6] But I am not writing this book for him; I am writing this book for my three sons and two daughters and all the children they will have. And I write for the sake of every child who will ever be born with the genetic patterns that make him or her susceptible to a form of rheumatoid disease.[7]

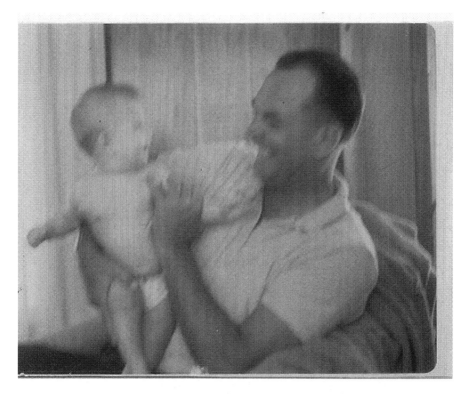

It is time that we ensure that they will not suffer as we did. We cannot wait for someone else to take the first step. Patients must be involved because it is our lives and our children's lives that are at stake. Patients are the only ones who fully know what living with this disease means.

I have told you part of my family's experience with rheumatoid disease, but the evidence that I present in this book is not from my personal experience or even that of other patients. It is evidence from medical literature. That evidence confirms the experience of millions of patients who know that "rheumatoid" is a disease.

This the right time for this change:

1) People with RD have come together for the first time in history through the Rheumatoid Patient Foundation.

2) Research has demonstrated the systemic nature of the disease, as we will see in the list of ten things that threaten patients' health.

3) Personalized medicine and collaboration with patients are now recognized as reasonable approaches to rheumatologic disease treatment,[8, 9] especially for a disease that is so heterogeneous.

This is a turning point. It is time to acknowledge and treat the whole disease. It is time to leave the misconceptions and myths about this disease in the past, along with the unfortunate inaccurate name "rheumatoid arthritis."

> "UNLESS WE PLAN ON CURING THESE TERRIBLE ILLNESSES IN THE NEAR FUTURE,
> I SUGGEST WE TAKE A SERIOUS LOOK AT HOW TO BEST INFORM THE PUBLIC AND
> THE ENTIRE HEALTHCARE ESTABLISHMENT OF THE INCREDIBLE SERIOUSNESS OF RHEUMATIC DISEASES,
> AND GET AS FAR AWAY AS POSSIBLE FROM A TRIVIAL CONCEPT OF 'ARTHRITIS.'"
>
> R. FRANKLIN ADAMS, M.D.

(Footnote.)[10]

A word to clinicians treating RD

As Dr. Adams illustrates in Chapter 7, you have a difficult and underappreciated job. Misunderstandings of RD have made medical diagnosis and treatment even more difficult. One goal of this book is to make your job easier and more successful. You will learn information that will expand, and sometimes even challenge what you have learned in school. If you do not have a close family member with RD, I hope you will imagine as you read that it is your mother or daughter or sibling or partner with this disease.

People with RD have suffered in many ways over the centuries, but one of the harshest ways has been the denial of extensive aspects of their illness. This has denied them appropriate treatment and contributed to premature death. But it has also harmed them by bringing unnecessary shame and guilt with insinuations that they are not as sick as they claim to be or that it is somehow their own fault, as Dr. Adams explains. Frequently accused of hypochondria and suspected of exaggeration, these patients have only wanted to be well and live out their lives. I hope the facts in this book will not only change minds but reach hearts. Let's change the way RD is regarded in the medical community.

A word to people living with RD

I know from my own story, and the stories of thousands of others, that you are living with the cruelest of conditions. It crushes you invisibly, steals more each day, and causes suffering that people without RD can never comprehend. If you have mild RD, I pray it never progresses to its full-blown state. Whether your RD is mild or severe, I hope you will use this book as your guide to get the best possible care for every danger of RD. It was difficult to write a book for you that can also be appreciated by the medical community, but it had to be done. So please don't let any medical lingo discourage you from learning about things you need to know. For simple definitions of abbreviations and terms, see the **Glossary and Tips** chapter at the back of this book.

We do not have all of the answers yet—like how to prevent this disease in our children or how to cure every danger it poses to our joints or organs. But I want you to keep in mind this one thing, that you deserve to be treated the same as any person without RD who faces any of these dangers. So, if you have lung symptoms, you deserve to be given the same tests and treatments as someone without RD who has those same lung problems. Nothing should be excused as "just" part of the RD. I know from experience that this is a supreme challenge. I know it's hard when a doctor doesn't know about problems caused by RD. Consider loaning this book to your doctor. Or write down the footnote reference and give her that. And I know it's so hard to see one more doctor or get one more scan. When you can't brush your hair, other problems like swollen lymph nodes can take a backseat. But you need to take the best care of yourself possible. You need to fight. You are warrior. You can do this.

---

[1] Johns Hopkins University [website]. Rheumatoid clip image 002 0005.jpg (image). 2011 Feb 17 [cited 2013 March 22]. Available from: http://vasculitis.med.jhu.edu/typesof/images/ rheumatoid_clip_image002_0005.jpg

[2] Immune suppression with methotrexate is defined by the CDC as 4 mg of methotrexate per kg of body weight per week (≤0.4 mg/kg/ week). Centers for Disease Control and Prevention [website]. 2011 Jan 28 [cited 2016 Mar 5]. Available from: http://www.cdc.gov/ mmwr/preview/mmwrhtml/rr6002a1.htm

[3] Young K. Doctors' understanding of rheumatoid disease does not align with patients' experiences. Brit Med J. 2013 May 14 [cited 2016 Feb 29];346:f2901. Available from: http://www.bmj.com/content/ 346/bmj.f2901 DOI: http://dx.doi.org/10.1136/bmj.f2901

[4] Rheumatoid Patient Foundation [website]. United States: c2011-2013 [cited 2013 Feb 20]. Available from: http:// rheum4us.org/

[5] Stuart G. Private world of pain. London: Allen and Unwin; 1953. 188 p.

[6] Young K. The tug of war of RA awareness: Privacy of pain & agony of disclosure. Rheumatoid Arthritis Warrior [website]. 2011 Mar 23 [cited 2016 May 31]. Available from: http://rawarrior.com/the-tug-of-war-of-ra-awareness-privacy-of-pain-agony-of-disclosure/

[7] Firestein GS. The disease formerly known as rheumatoid arthritis. Arthritis Res Ther. 2014 Jun 26 [cited 2016 Mar 5];16:114. Available from: http://arthritis-research.biomedcentral.com/articles/10.1186/ar4593 DOI: 10.1186/ar4593

[8] Colmegna I, Ohata BR, Menard HA. Current understanding of rheumatoid arthritis therapy. Clin Pharmacol Ther. 2012 [cited 2013 Mar 23];91(4):607-620. DOI:10.1038/clpt.2011.325

[9] van Tuyl LHD, Boers M. Patient's global assessment of Disease activity: What are we measuring? Arthritis Rheum. 2012 Sep [cited 2016 Feb 29];64(9):2811–2813 DOI: 10.1002/art.34540

[10] Adams RF. An identity crisis for RA: A few suggestions to bring rheumatic disease the recognition and respect it deserves. Atlanta (GA): American College of Rheumatology. The Rheumatologist. 2011 Aug 14 [cited 2012 Jul 20]. Available from: http://www.the-rheumatologist.org/details/article/1311755/An_Identity_Crisis_for_RA.html

CHAPTER ONE
WHAT IS RA REALLY?

Modernizing the label rheumatoid arthritis (RA) to the historic term rheumatoid disease (RD)

A new name for RA that's actually old: RD

If it's true that rheumatoid disease is not a form of arthritis, but a complex disease that can present many dangers to a person's health, then what should be done differently? Could people be diagnosed earlier or treated differently if this were readily recognized? Does it make any difference?

These are questions to bear in mind as we examine the evidence of the dangers of rheumatoid disease. I believe there have been grave consequences to perpetuating the misnomer of "arthritis." In fact, acknowledging that RD is not a form of arthritis is possibly the one action that could make the most impact on the major health threats faced by people living with RD. Let us look carefully at the nature of RA/RD, and consider how best to protect patients' health in light of the *10 Dangers of Rheumatoid Disease* outlined ahead.

Two notions of the systemic nature of this disease

RD is a systemic disease. This is something no one with

medical knowledge disputes. But, what does that imply? To those who live with the disease and a few who study it specifically, the phrase *systemic disease* has one meaning with regard to RD. It represents a long-term illness that causes systemic problems, which can be expressed in a variety of ways, including

> 1) **constitutional symptoms** like fatigue, dry eyes, vasculitis, low appetite, or fever

> 2) a myriad of **musculoskeletal conditions** such as synovitis, bursitis, Baker's cysts, tenosynovitis, or bone erosion, and symptoms like stiffness, weakness, and pain

> 3) **extra-articular disease**, organ conditions such as ischemic lung disease, pericarditis, or Still's disease. As a Johns Hopkins Hospital doctor wrote, "rheumatoid arthritis should be viewed as a multi-system disease affecting multiple organs."[1]

What else could *systemic disease* mean? In recent decades, the term "systemic disease" has been perfunctorily included in many descriptions of RA, without any reference to the many medical consequences such as those listed above. So, what does "systemic disease" mean to most people? It means that there is a systemic aspect to the disease so that RA may spread throughout the body to affect new joints. It is routinely, yet incorrectly, maintained that although the disease is considered "systemic" and treatments are administered systemically (by pills or shots), RA usually only attacks synovial joint tissue.

WHAT RD IS NOT

1. RD is unrelated to the process usually referred to as "arthritis," a degeneration of joint cartilage commonly occurring in athletes due to over-use or in most adults as a result of the normal process of aging. This is often referred to as osteoarthritis (OA), in an attempt to minimize confusion between arthritis and disease processes such as RA. OA is extremely common, eventually occurring to some degree in virtually everyone. Although OA is even more common in people who have RD, RD is not a type of OA and is unrelated to OA.

2. RD is not caused by lifestyle choices like poor diet, lack of exercise, or having a bad temperament. Old theories of rheumatoid personality,[2] in which RD is blamed on feelings about one's mother or an inflexible attitude[3, 4] or other theories linking RD to major depression have been disproven.[5, 6] Although tobacco smoking has been associated with a higher incidence of RD, millions have been diagnosed with RD without ever having smoked. No explicit causative factors of RD have been identified. You can't "do" something to prevent RD. Centuries of faulty theories about this subject have contributed to the stigma and "taboo"[7, 8] related to RD in some cultures. This is most obviously undeserved by children with the disease.

Media articles often warn that RD can be caused or worsened by inadequate physical activity; however, research has shown that the risk of RD is actually greater in people who have a history of a higher level of physical activity.[9] Likewise, medical websites present an almost universal refrain with regard to weight loss, asserting that being overweight is a cause of RA or RA severity. However low body weight has been shown to be a significant indicator of more severe rheumatoid disease[10] and worse outcomes.[11] Weight loss and lower BMI are in fact predictive of death in RD.[12] (Increased weight or reduced exercise can certainly occur with RD for various medical reasons including effects of the disease and medications.)

3. RD is not a hand disease. Until new criteria were adopted in 2010,[13] diagnosis of rheumatoid arthritis required visibly detectable swelling in hand joints, including fingers or wrists, as one of the necessary symptoms. The newer guidelines continue to dramatically emphasize swelling of the small joints of the hands and feet and fail to consider other symptoms.

Conspicuous swelling of hand joints is also the primary gauge of disease activity for many rheumatologists, judging by interviews with several doctors and comments from many patients. Patients often experience remarks such as these: "My rheumatologist bases my RA activity solely on swollen joints of my hands"[14] and "Doc told me the only joints that the RA would cause pain in is the small joints of the hands and feet."[15] The conception of RA as "a type of arthritis" contributes to the hand disease model. One consequence of the hand disease / arthritis perception is incomplete measurement of disease activity, both articular (of the joints) and extra-articular (non-joint).

Emphasis on hands in the diagnosis and evaluation of RD is the result of a persistent myth that RA affects the hands or small joints first and worst. The assumption is accepted almost universally in medical settings. However, the first RD symptom experienced by patients may actually be in any joint or it may be one of many non-joint symptoms,[16] as thousands of patients in our RD community have testified. In some patients, hands are the first affected area, but this is not always the case, as seen in 880 patient comments on one article.[17] In different sections of this book, you will also read several investigators' statements about various extra-articular features appearing as the first RD symptom, including lung and blood vessel involvement.

1ST SYMPTOM OF RA
Responses from >880 patients

Feet	Heart	Eyes (uveitis, scleritis, iritis)
Shoulder	Fever	High ESR (sed rate)
Back / spine / neck	Knee	Digestive inflammation
Hip	Jaw	Flu symptoms
Hand	Fatigue	Skin rash
Ankle	Vasculitis	Nodule
All joints at once	Sternum	Weight loss
SI joint	Elbow	Lung (sarcoidosis, inflammation)
Wrist	Bone pain	

WHAT RD IS

1. RD is an inflammatory disease that causes systemic illness and frequently affects joints in a symmetrical pattern. Most prominently, it can cause severe pain, sudden functional loss, and ultimately lead to destruction of tissues related to joints. Other common symptoms include fatigue, fever, stiffness, swelling, and weakness. The disease can cause problems with various organs or systems, including the circulatory or nervous systems, eyes, skin, heart, or lungs.[18] As expert rheumatologist Joan Bathon points out, "It can be in all your tissues, causing problems wherever inflammation occurs."[19] Daniel Arkfeld, a rheumatologist at the University of Southern California's Keck Medical Center, explains it this way: "I think it's important to understand that rheumatoid arthritis comes from the blood... And it's a trafficking of immune factors in the blood that go to the joints. The disease doesn't start in the joints; it's really in the blood."[20]

Cardiovascular and lung disease have sometimes been viewed

as co-morbidities to RD; however, a more accurate understanding is that they are *involvement of the disease itself*.[21] Recent investigation shows that rheumatoid disease may be present prior to articular manifestations that are diagnosable as RD,[22] which has given rise to the term "pre-clinical RA."[23] Mayo Clinic's consistent reporting of the persistent mortality gap in RD[24] has led to examination of its causes, which are often heart or lung related.[25, 26]

2. RD is a chronic immune system disruption. The prevalent belief has been that in the presence of particular alleles (genetic components), some sort of environmental trigger initiates a lasting autoimmune response. Autoimmunity is understood as one's immune system attacking one's own tissues, as evidenced by the existence of particular antibodies such as rheumatoid factors or antibodies to cyclic citrullinated peptides (anti-CCP). Examination of excess immune activity is an extremely fertile research area, as many diseases seem to be linked to immune activity. No one knows exactly how it begins or how to stop it.

That lack of explanation, along with mediocre success in treating the disease, has fueled continued investigation of the origin of diseases like RA that are believed to be "autoimmune." One crucial problem that must be addressed is the diversity with regard to the presence of antibodies found in individual patients with obvious evidence of the disease. Even the basic notions of autoimmunity could be suspect, at least in cases where antibodies are not found.

One emerging scenario considers whether the presence of microbes on mucosal surfaces (such as lungs or mouth) leads to inflammatory activity, possibly reviving previous theories of infectious causes to RD.[27] The current model of autoimmunity has come into question as evidence continues to mount of a connection between microorganisms and immune-mediated diseases. "The practice of rheumatology has assumed that in 'nonseptic' inflammatory disorders, the immune response is an over-reaction. Could it instead represent a deficiency in the host's ability to clear microorganisms?"[28] This remains to be seen with further investigation of the microbiome.

However, much more research has been directed toward exploring causes for the "loss of tolerance" to self and the initiation of autoimmunity in diseases like RD.

For example, the role of human endogenous retroviruses (HERVs) has been investigated for implications relating to the initiation of the disease. In a review of nearly one hundred papers, Tugnet et al. found "The evidence appears to be mounting for HERV-K10 in RA pathogenesis."[29] HERVs reverse the normal flow of genetic information from DNA to RNA, known as "reverse transcription," and since they are transmitted genetically, they are considered trapped within the human genome. HERVs could be a mechanism in setting the genetic stage for autoimmunity according to several hypotheses.

3. RD is broadly heterogeneous. The course of the disease varies between patients, and vexingly, in the same patient over time. Similarly, response to treatment is unpredictable in a particular patient, varies between patients, and fluctuates over time. "Overall, heterogeneity of treatment effect is the result of the relative dominance of one biological pathway over others in a particular individual, and the dominant pathway may vary in a given patient during the course of the disease."[30]

RD may be viewed as a syndrome with several identifiable subsets.[31] Categories could be created according to presence of antibodies, particular alleles, or other markers. So, "...a molecular taxonomy for 'the rheumatoid arthritis syndrome' is feasible. Patients with ACPA-positive (anti-CCP) disease have a less favorable prognosis than those with ACPA-negative disease, which suggests that such molecular subsets are clinically useful."[32]

Some have begun to view RD as a group of diseases that, while similar, may more successfully be treated when identified separately.[33] The suggestion was made as early as 1960 to separate rheumatoid cases into phenotypes, according to similarity of disease course.[34] The simplest answer to the question "what is RD?" is also the most extraordinary: it is a mysterious disease. As much we have learned in recent years about rheumatoid disease, it is unknown exactly what it is or how it can be stopped.

A noun tells what something is

Author and activist e-Patient Dave deBronkart plainly stated the source of disconnect in the minds of people in most discussions of "rheumatoid arthritis": "Rheumatoid is an adjective; applied to 'arthritis' people hear it as 'arthritis, a particular kind of arthritis.'"[35] Of course, the noun is always the most fundamental item in any communication. While a turkey sandwich may vary greatly from a cheese sandwich, in either case it is obvious that, indisputably, the essential theme is food —and specifically, food served on two pieces of bread. And just as someone might subsequently refer to his "sandwich" instead of his "cheese," a "particular type of arthritis" becomes synonymous with the term "arthritis."

It's logical that once RA is labeled as "a type of arthritis," it gets abbreviated to "arthritis." Evidence of Dave's point is seen in the way people, including medical professionals and journalists, frequently abbreviate the term "rheumatoid arthritis" to just "arthritis."[36, 37, 38] The word "arthritis" is often used to refer to RA in all types of mass media, as well as educational meetings, general medical settings, and clinical environments. Regular instances of this interchangeability demonstrate the confusion of the public created as a result.[39, 40, 41] Patients' frustration about these articles is palpable.[42, 43, 44] In Chapter 12, you'll read about how this confusion also interferes with the accurate collection or reporting of data.

Correctly framing the dangers of RD

Accurate language is obviously essential to communication. Medical terms should not only be well defined, but also reliably convey a reality. Lupus or systemic lupus erythematosus (SLE), for example, is a similar disease to rheumatoid disease. While symptoms of lupus include joint inflammation, the disease has not been called "lupus arthritis."

Undeniably, perceptions of RD have been distorted by the label of "arthritis."

This book will demonstrate the fallacy of labeling rheumatoid disease as one of its symptoms, arthritis, and thereby limiting the perception of the disease to that one symptom. Joint inflammation (arthritis) is one overt and often devastating symptom of RD. But unfortunately, it is not the only symptom. It is not the one that shortens lives. And, importantly, arthritis does not appear to be the earliest medical indication of RD, so using it as the sole diagnostic criterion does not provide for the earliest possible diagnosis and treatment.

Despite what patients are commonly told and what is commonly taught in medical contexts, it is not rare for RD to impact a patient's health beyond the joints. To the contrary, it appears to be universal. This book will outline ten specific perils to living with RD—***10 Dangers of Rheumatoid Disease***. These are areas of which people with RD need to be aware, consider taking precautions, and possibly pursue medical treatment.

This book will also highlight reasons for using a more accurate label for this dangerous disease, how that change benefits doctors as well as patients and those who care for them. We will learn from patients, researchers, and clinicians about the advantages to updating the language. We will see how a fairly easy change could have significant impact on the lives of millions of people.

*For a handy reference of what is RD and what is not, see the **Glossary & Tips** chapter at the back of this book.*

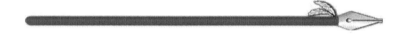

KEY POINTS

1. Saying RD is a systemic disease does not just mean it spreads systemically. RD causes systemic illness that can show up in these ways:

    a. Constitutional symptoms like fatigue, fever, or dry eyes

    b. Musculoskeletal conditions such as synovitis, bursitis, Baker's cysts, tenosynovitis, or bone erosion, and symptoms like stiffness, weakness, and pain

    c. Organ conditions such as ischemic lung disease, pericarditis, or Still's disease, and many others discussed in this book

2. The "hand disease" model is part of the "type of arthritis" model. It's wrong. RD does not start in the hands and they are not always an accurate reflection of disease activity.

3. RD is an immune disruption caused by genetic influence and possible environmental triggers.

4. RD is very heterogeneous.

5. Arthritis is only one symptom of RD. It's usually the most obvious symptom, but not the one that shortens lives.

Action step: Don't assume that hand or joint symptoms are the best indication of rheumatoid disease activity. Investigate and treat extra-articular symptoms of RD.

Quote to remember: Undeniably, perceptions of rheumatoid disease (RD) have been distorted by the label "rheumatoid arthritis."

---

[1] Pappas D. Lung involvement in patients with rheumatoid arthritis. The Johns Hopkins Arthritis Center [website]. 2012 Mar 27 [cited 2013 Mar 23]. Available from http://www.hopkinsarthritis.org/arthritis-info/rheumatoid-arthritis/lung-involvement-in-ra/

[2] Arthritis Foundation. Good living with rheumatoid arthritis. 3rd ed. Atlanta (GA); 2006. 299 p.

[3] Chopra D. Ageless body, timeless mind: The quantum alternative to growing old, p 66. NY: Three Rivers Press; 1993. ISBN: 978-0-517-88212-2. 342 p.

[4] Segal I. The secret language of your body: The essential guide to

health and wellness, p 140: Victoria, Australia: Blue Angel Gallery; 2007. 216 p.

[5] Yamanaka H, Seto Y, Tanaka E, Furuya T, Nakajima A, Ikari K, Taniguchi A, Momohara S. Management of rheumatoid arthritis: The 2012 perspective. Mod Rheumatol. 2013 Jan 23 [cited 2013 Mar 12]; (1):1-7. Available from: http://www.ncbi.nlm.nih.gov/pubmed/22772460 DOI: 10.1007/s10165-012-0702-1

[6] Pincus T, Callahan LF, Bradley LA, Vaughn WK, Wolfe F. Elevated MMPI scores for hypochondriasis, depression, and hysteria in patients with rheumatoid arthritis reflect disease rather than psychological status. Arthritis Rheum. 1986 Dec [cited 2012 Sep 30]; 29(12):1456-66. Available from: http://onlinelibrary.wiley.com/store/10.1002/art.1780291206/asset/1780291206_ftp.pdf?v=1&t=heygbmmo&s=51c87757d57a692e9eb1e9d28b6a59c81651c5c4

[7] Preethi, an RA patient. In: Young K. Sympathy and living with rheumatoid arthritis symptoms. Rheumatoid Arthritis Warrior [website]. 2010 Dec 19 [cited 2013 Mar 23]. Available from: http://rawarrior.com/sympathy-and-living-with-rheumatoid-arthritis-symptoms/?show=comments#comment-45983

[8] Young K. Rheumatoid arthritis disease may be the scarlet RA. Rheumatoid Arthritis Warrior [website]. 2009 Dec 11 [cited 2017 Jun 17]. http://rawarrior.com/rheumatoid-arthritis-disease-may-be-the-scarlet-ra/

[9] Zeng P, Klareskog L, Alfredsson L, Bengtsson C. Physical workload is associated with increased risk of rheumatoid arthritis: Results from a Swedish population-based case–control study. RMD Open. 2017 Mar 14 [cited 2017 Jun 17];3(1):e000324. Available from: http://rmdopen.bmj.com/content/3/1/e000324. DOI: 10.1136/rmdopen-2016-000324

[10] Fleming A, Crown JM, Corbett M. Prognostic value of early features in rheumatoid disease. Br Med J. 1976 May 22 [cited 2017 Jul 8]; 1(6020):1243-5. Available from: https://www.ncbi.nlm.nih.gov/pmc/articles/PMC1639812/

[11] Fleming A, Dodman S, Crown JM, Corbett M. Extra-articular features in early rheumatoid disease. Brit Med J. 1976 May 22 [cited 2013 Apr 20];1:1241-1243. Available from: http://www.ncbi.nlm.nih.gov/pmc/articles/PMC1639805/pdf/brmedj00517-0011.pdf

[12] Baker JF, Billig E, Michaud K, Ibrahim S, Caplan L, Cannon GW, Stokes A, Majithia V, Mikuls TR. Weight loss, the obesity paradox, and the risk of death in rheumatoid arthritis. Arthrit Rheum. 2015 [cited 2017 Jun 17]67:1711–1717. DOI:10.1002/art.39136

[13] Aletaha D, Neogi T, Silman AJ, Funovits J, Felson DT, Bingham CO, Birnbaum NS, Burmester GR, Bykerk VP, Cohen MD, et al. 2010 Rheumatoid arthritis classification criteria: An American College of Rheumatology/European League Against Rheumatism collaborative initiative. Arthritis Rheum. 2010 Sep [cited 2013 Feb 23];62(9): 2569–2581. Available from: http://onlinelibrary.wiley.com/doi/10.1002/art.27584/full doi: 10.1002/art.27584

[14] Marianne, an RA patient. In: Young K. A paradigm shift in rheumatoid arthritis disease activity? Part 2. Rheumatoid Arthritis Warrior [website]. 2011 Oct 15 [cited 2013 Mar 23]. Available from: http://rawarrior.com/a-paradigm-shift-in-rheumatoid-arthritis-disease-activity-part-2/?show=comments#comment-101341

[15] Nancy, an RA patient. In: Young K. "Inadequate & stupid? No, just a victim of someone's training". Rheumatoid Arthritis Warrior [website]. 2013 Jun 28 [cited 2017 Jun 17]. Available from: http://rawarrior.com/inadequate-stupid-no-just-a-victim-of-someones-training/

[16] Young K. 15 Early Symptoms of Rheumatoid Arthritis. Rheumatoid Arthritis Warrior [website]. 2016 Feb 4 [cited 2016 Feb 28]. Available from: http://rawarrior.com/15-early-symptoms-of-rheumatoid-arthritis/

[17] RA patients. What is the first symptom of rheumatoid arthritis? Rheumatoid Arthritis Warrior [website]. 2009 [cited 2016 Feb 28]. Available from: http://rawarrior.com/what-is-

the-first-symptom-of-rheumatoid-arthritis/?show=comments

[18] McInnes IB, Schett G. The pathogenesis of rheumatoid arthritis. New Engl J Med. 2011 Dec 8 [cited 2013 Jan 24];365:2205-2219. Available from: http://www.nejm.org/doi/pdf/10.1056/NEJMra1004965 DOI: 10.1056/NEJMra1004965

[19] Abedin S. 10 serious RA symptoms to never ignore: There's more than joint pain to watch out for. WebMD [website]. 2011 Jan 12 [cited 2013 Mar 23]. Available from: http://www.webmd.com/rheumatoid-arthritis/features/10-serious-rheumatoid-arthritis-symptoms

[20] Martinez J. Doctor, patients: Rheumatoid arthritis is far more than joint pain. Southern California Public Radio Blogs [website]. 2013 Feb 4 [cited 2013 Mar 30]. Available from: http://www.scpr.org/blogs/southla/2013/02/04/12345/doctor-patients-rheumatoid-arthritis-far-more-join/

[21] Bands A. Extra-articular lesions of rheumatoid arthritis. Brit Med J. 1973 Sep 29 [cited 2013 Apr 21]. Available from: http://europepmc.org/articles/PMC1587013/pdf/brmedj01577-0017a.pdf

[22] Fischer A, Solomon JJ, du Bois RM, Deane KD, Olson AL, Fernandez-Perez ER, Huie TJ, Stevens AD, Gill MB, Rabinovitch AM, et al. Lung disease with anti-CCP antibodies but not rheumatoid arthritis or connective tissue disease. Resp Med. 2012 Jul [cited 2013 Mar 23];106(7):1040-1047. Available from: http://

www.ncbi.nlm.nih.gov/pubmed/22503074. DOI: 10.1016/j.rmed.
2012.03.006

[23] Young K. Preclinical rheumatoid disease: There are no joints in the lungs. Rheumatoid Arthritis Warrior [website]. 2012 Mar 18 [cited 2013 Mar 23]. Available from: http://rawarrior.com/preclinical-rheumatoid-disease-there-are-no-joints-in-the-lungs

[24] Gonzalez A, Maradit Kremers H, Crowson CS, Nicola P J, Davis JM, Therneau TM, Roger VL, Gabriel SE. The widening mortality gap between rheumatoid arthritis patients and the general population. Arthritis Rheum. 2007 Nov [cited 2013 Mar 23];56: 3583–3587. Available from: http://onlinelibrary.wiley.com/doi/10.1002/art.22979/full DOI: 10.1002/art.22979

[25] Gabriel SE. Why do people with rheumatoid arthritis still die prematurely? Ann Rheum Dis. 2008 Jul 10 [cited Mar 23];67:Suppl 3 iii30-iii34. Available from: http://ard.bmj.com/content/67/Suppl_3/iii30.full

[26] Tsuchiya Y, Takayanagi N, Sugiura H, Miyahara Y, Tokunaga D, Kawabata Y, Sugita Y. Lung diseases directly associated with rheumatoid arthritis and their relationship to outcome. Eur Respir J. 2011 Jun 1 [cited 2013 Mar 23];37(6):1411-1417. Available from: http://erj.ersjournals.com/content/37/6/1411.long

[27] Deane K, Mikuls T. Preventing rheumatoid arthritis? The links to mucosa. Musculoskeletal Network [website]. 2013 Jan 14 [cited 2013 Mar 23]. Available from: http://www.musculoskeletalnetwork.com/rheumatoid-arthritis/content/article/1145622/2122794

[28] Paget S. The microbiome and autoimmunity: Seven signs of impending paradigm change. Musculoskeletal Network [website]. 2013 Mar 19 [cited 2013 Mar 22]. Available from: http://www.musculoskeletalnetwork.com/rheumatic-diseases/content/article/1145622/2133513

[29] Tugnet N, Rylance P, Roden D, Trela M, Nelson P. Human endogenous retroviruses (HERVs) and autoimmune rheumatic disease: Is there a link? Open Rheumatol J. 2013 Mar 22 [cited 2017 Mar 24];7:13–21. Available from: https://www.ncbi.nlm.nih.gov/pmc/articles/PMC3636489/

[30] Colmegna et al. Current understanding of rheumatoid arthritis therapy. (See footnote in Introduction.)

[31] Chemin K, Klareskog L, Malmstrom V. Is rheumatoid arthritis an autoimmune disease? Curr Opin Rheumatol. 2016 Mar [cited 2016 Feb 28];28(2):181-8. DOI:1 0.1 097/BOR.0000000000000253

[32] McInnes IB. The pathogenesis of rheumatoid arthritis. (See footnote Introduction.)

[33] Shammas RM, Ranganath VK, Paulus HE. Remission in rheumatoid arthritis. Curr Rheumatol Rep. 2010 Oct [cited 2013 Mar 23];12(5):355–362. Available from: http://www.ncbi.nlm.nih.gov/pmc/articles/PMC2927687/

[34] Jonsson E. On the prognosis of rheumatoid arthritis. Acta orthopaedica Scandinavica. Stoholm (Sweden): The Medical Department III, South Hospital. 1960 [cited 2013 Mar 23];30:115-23. Available from: http://www.ncbi.nlm.nih.gov/pubmed/13790644

[35] deBronkart D, Comment in: Young K. Will Venus Williams' Sjögren's syndrome help RA? Rheumatoid Arthritis Warrior [website]. 2011 Sep 2 [cited 2013 Mar 23]. Available from: http://rawarrior.com/will-venus-williams-sjogrens-syndrome-help-ra/?show=comments#comment-88827

[36] Zoler ML. PAD prevalent in arthritis patients. Rheumatology News [website]. 2009 Aug [cited 2013 Apr 27]:28. Available from: http://www.acssurgerynews.com/fileadmin/content_pdf/rheum/archive_pdf/vol8iss8/70244_main.pdf

[37] Illinois Department of Health [website]. Rheumatoid arthritis and heart disease. 2008 May 8 [cited 2013 Apr 28]. Available from: http://www.idph.state.il.us/about/chronic/ra_cvd_fs.htm

[38] Lutz R. Arthritis drugs for the treatment of vitiligo. MD Magazine [website]. 2015 Nov 5 [cited 2017 Jul 9]. Available from: http://www.mdmag.com/medical-news/arthritis-drugs-for-the-treatment-of-vitiligo

[39] Clark L. Arthritis symptoms: Seven signs you could be suffering with painful condition. Daily Express [website]. 2017 Apr 21 [cited 2017 Jun 17]. Available from: http://www.express.co.uk/life-style/health/794768/arthritis-rheumatoid-osteoarthritis-joints-symptoms

[40] Daily Journal [website]. Health lines: Arthritis common condition, but not easily understood by all. 2017 Apr 14 [cited 2017 Jun 17]. Available from: http://www.djournal.com/lifestyle/health/health-lines-arthritis-common-condition-but-not-easily-understood-by/article_a23b9151-8260-5ca5-9dd9-a40910faf36e.html

[41] Sunrise Senior Living [website]. Spotting chronic conditions: 6 ways to manage arthritis pain. 2017 Apr 5 [cited 2017 Jun 17]. Available from: https://www.sunriseseniorliving.com/blog/april-2017/spotting-chronic-conditions-6-ways-to-manage-arthritis-pain.aspx

[42] RA patients. RA Warrior Facebook Page. Facebook [website]. 2017 Apr 24 [cited 2017 Jun 17]. Available from https://www.facebook.com/arthritiswarrior/posts/10155041973985726

[43] RA patients. RA Warrior Facebook Page. Facebook [website]. 2017 Apr 20 [cited 2017 Jun 17]. Available from https://www.facebook.com/arthritiswarrior/posts/10155018991940726

[44] RA patients. RA Warrior Facebook Page. Facebook [website]. 2017 Apr 14 [cited 2017 Jun 17]. Available from: https://

www.facebook.com/arthritiswarrior/posts/10154991173175726

CHAPTER TWO
IMPACT OF THE MASK

How the "arthritis" mask contributes to the dangers of rheumatoid disease

Managing the disease in the midst of misconceptions

This chapter presents a brief look at specific ways the mask of arthritis can affect diagnosis and treatment of rheumatoid disease as well as provoke misunderstanding in real-life circumstances. For people living with rheumatoid disease (PRD), the dangers of the disease discussed in future chapters usually exist behind that mask and within the context of these misunderstandings. No doubt the consequences of these dangers intensify when we ignore the dangers themselves, since they lurk behind a label of "arthritis."

Someday, the problem of rheumatoid disease (RD) will be solved by the simple fact of a cure. Until that day, three common problems plague people with RD. Each of these persistent issues is related in part to the mistaken notion of RA as a "type of arthritis."

> "WE MUST FACE THE REALITY THAT
> ANYTHING WITH 'ARTHRITIS' AS PART OF ITS NAME
> IS LIKELY TO BE RELEGATED
> TO A SECOND TIER OF HUMAN SUFFERING."
>
> R. FRANKLIN ADAMS, M.D.

(Footnote.)[1]

PROBLEM ONE: The lack of effective treatments for various aspects of the disease

Joint symptoms

Current disease treatments are highly effective at reducing joint symptoms for only a minority of patients. Even in clinical trials with carefully chosen patients who are provided optimal care, only 20% of patients generally experience 70 percent improvement.[2] Reliably, studies show one-third of patients to be non-responsive to currently available disease treatments. Fewer than half of patients experience 50 percent improvement of symptoms.[3]

While a small number of European investigators have better results in aggressive treatment of exclusive "very-early" or pre-clinical RA populations, the rate of joint symptom-based remission in the United States (U.S.) remains low, reported at about six percent.[4] Most patients continue to experience joint symptoms despite treatment, and it is difficult for clinicians to quantify joint symptoms over time. PRD also treat symptoms with anti-inflammatories like steroids and NSAIDs, pain medications, and alternative methods like compression, ice or heat packs, and massage. PRD experience a range of joint symptoms during the three to six months between rheumatology appointments. These symptoms are impossible for clinicians to gauge by visible assessment of swelling in a single moment.

Although most rheumatologists rate disease activity by conspicuous swelling,[5] joint symptoms are actually not limited to visible swelling, and swelling does not perfectly correlate with other joint symptoms. Swelling does not always associate with damage either. Seventy-five percent of patients surveyed experienced either swelling without damage or had damage occur without any obvious swelling.[6]

Investigators are finding biomarkers such as the 14-3-3eta protein that do not always correlate with inflammation measures or other recognized rheumatoid antibodies, but nonetheless correlate with damage in RA.[7] If damage and inflammation are two separate symptoms in RA, and if different proteins have different roles in the rheumatoid disease process, then it is logical that damage in joints does not always correlate with obvious swelling. (See also discussion of ACPA's role, Chapter 3, "Recent advances in understanding rheumatoid disease.")

PRD experience an array of joint symptoms other than swelling which are usually not considered. Pain is the most significant way in which a patient is aware of disease activity in a joint, but PRD mention other symptoms including stiffness, weakness, tenderness, warmth, twisting or unnatural positioning, burning, numbness, redness, a tearing sensation, and loss of dexterity or agility.

Several lesser-known joints are commonly affected by the disease, but receive very little attention because they do not fit the current arthritis paradigm for the disease. The cricoarytenoid joints are cartilage joints in the larynx, which are used during speech. When they are inflamed or stiffened, the voice can become hoarse or a PRD can have difficulty breathing. The cartilage joints where the ribs meet the sternum also often remain inflamed (costochondritis) despite treatment even when more obvious joints seem quiet.

Extra-articular disease effects

Most rheumatoid patients must manage a range of extra-articular disease symptoms that are not usually monitored or treated by rheumatologists. Constitutional effects of the disease that may persist despite treatment include fatigue, fever, and skin symptoms such as nodules, redness, or rashes. Some PRD also experience loss of appetite, weakness, or a flu-like sense of being unwell, likely as a result of persistent disease activity.

The systemic inflammation and destructive immune activity of RD can also result in various types of damage to vital organs including the lungs and heart.[8] Several types of cardiovascular and lung disease occur as direct extra-articular results of the disease. Evidence is somewhat encouraging yet inconsistent as to whether currently available treatments help to reduce the systemic toll of the disease or whether they improve mortality.[9] [10] [11] [12]

Other systemic problems can occur as a direct result of RD, including Sjögren's syndrome, anemia, vasculitis, and Still's disease. In spite of reduced hand swelling, constitutional symptoms, spine problems, or extra-articular manifestations often continue to contribute to worsening health or disability. Inflammation of spinal joints also leads to problems in arms and legs such as sciatica, neuropathy, or more critical problems. A dangerously unstable cervical spine must be recognized so life-saving measures can be taken.[13] [14]

Note: This book will treat comorbidities as a separate category from extra-articular disease because comorbidities are not a direct result of RD. The Key Points summary at the end of this chapter has an easy list of these categories. It can be difficult to separate them since many physicians and researchers use the terms interchangeably. Examples of common comorbidities include Type 1 diabetes, thyroid disease, and celiac disease. These will not be considered among the distinct dangers of RD.

Impact on disease management

After over a decade of use and two decades of research, success rates of modern treatments remain mediocre because researchers—like clinicians—still rely mostly upon visible joint symptoms as the principal gauge of disease activity for a systemic disease that can affect nearly any organ or part of the body. Current diagnostic criteria and measures of disease activity do not take constitutional symptoms or other extra-articular disease manifestations into account.

One unfortunate effect of viewing the disease solely in terms of joint symptoms is the undocumented smoldering disease activity that takes place even in so-called responders to treatment. Nearly every patient I've met who has been told she is "in remission" experiences joint symptoms either regularly or in the form of periodic flares. Furthermore, I have observed numerous PRD who experienced serious extra-articular illness after long periods of treatment-induced joint-symptom "remission."

Investigators are also finding that extra-articular disease is significant, even if joint symptoms seem to be subdued. An editorial by Harvard rheumatology investigator Daniel Solomon points out that even when medical treatment successfully improves joint symptoms, "patients with RA continue to suffer from a variety of extra-articular manifestations, including cardiovascular disease (CVD)."[15] Yunt and Solomon also found that "control of joint disease does not translate to control of lung disease" in people with RD.[16] Researchers are even working in labs to create better models for investigating RD (see Chapters 3 and 5) that include more of the extra-articular disease than the current models that are used to induce joint symptoms in mice such as CIA (collagen-induced arthritis).

Health care professionals are mainly aware that the disease affects hands, but other disease symptoms are less readily acknowledged, examined, or measured. While the disease is referred to as "a type of arthritis,"[17] it is difficult for PRD to obtain appropriate medical attention for non-joint symptoms or for lesser-known "joints" such as vocal cords. Effective treatments do not yet exist to eliminate every disease effect in every patient. However, making clinicians, academics, and investigators aware of systemic disease effects is a necessary first step.

> "THE WIDESPREAD SYSTEMIC NATURE OF
> CERTAIN CASES OF RHEUMATOID ARTHRITIS HAS BEEN NOTED.
> IT IS SUGGESTED THAT 'RHEUMATOID DISEASE'
> IS A PREFERABLE TERM
> WHOSE PRINCIPAL CLINICAL MANIFESTATION IS 'ARTHRITIS'..."
> 1948 ELLMAN & BALL, BRITISH MEDICAL JOURAL

(Footnote.)[18]

PROBLEM TWO: Inadequate assistance or accommodation

An almost universal occurrence for people living with rheumatoid disease is that others confuse the disease with "arthritis," also referred to as "osteoarthritis" or OA. This confusion results in skepticism about the seriousness of RD and a decreased likelihood that a PRD will receive necessary accommodations in either occupational or social circumstances.

Work circumstances

Work disability remains high for PRD, with studies estimating at least a third cannot work after two to ten years disease duration, and with the percentage climbing in longer standing disease.[19, 20] Even in the decade of the 2000's with the most modern treatments, 20% of newly diagnosed patients who were working when diagnosed are work disabled after two years and 32% after five years.[21] Work disability has been viewed for decades as an additional aspect of the burden on PRD.

It is likely that some PRD could continue to work with accommodations related to schedules, shifts, and physical position or location of work. Many PRD experience a dramatic flaring pattern of disease that is unfamiliar to non-PRD and not easily relatable to "arthritis." Early work cessation rates could be reduced with improved understanding of the disease experience, as well as other flexible practices such as allowing patients to better manage days missed for medical treatment or other disease consequences.

People are often unaware that their expectations of PRD are unreasonable because symptoms are not usually visibly obvious. Employers may assume that if RA is "a form of arthritis," it does not warrant widespread accommodations. For example, patients report being asked to refrain from using a reserved handicapped parking space at work despite being legally entitled to do so, as long as there is a state-issued permit displayed in the car. [22, 23, 24]

Accommodation for all types of conditions improves as public awareness increases. More accurate language will result in improved workplace awareness of the complexity of rheumatoid disease, and it will possibly help PRD to remain employed longer. PRD rank supportive colleagues and managers as important factors in remaining employed.[25]

Personal and social circumstances

Confusion about RD results in a lack of the kind of social support that frequently exists for other comparable diseases like type 1 diabetes (T1D) or multiple sclerosis (MS). Many people with RD report having received much greater levels of assistance within their personal sphere when experiencing better understood illnesses such as a sprained ankle or gall bladder surgery.

PRD may not be able to fulfill usual family responsibilities on a regular basis without assistance. They may need more support than they appear to need since symptoms of the disease often are not obvious. This further confuses those who consider the disease to be similar to the "regular arthritis" which most people experience to some degree. The experience of living with RD is not comparable to having arthritis, and the difference is not one of degree.

Living with RD, a chronic progressive systemic disease, is more like living with type 1 diabetes or MS than it is like having arthritis. PRD may need assistance with personal care or family responsibilities, they need may help with shopping or getting to frequent medical appointments, and they need understanding related to persistent pain, extensive medications, unfamiliar symptoms, and numerous medical procedures due to disease progression.

Relationships that should be a wealth of needed support are often affected adversely. Both men and women with PRD frequently report that others are unable to accept (1) needs related to the illness, or (2) an inability to fulfill expected roles. Conflicts are often rooted in misperceptions created by the use of the word "arthritis." I've received hundreds of messages from patients who tell similar stories about the way others respond to them as soon as the word "arthritis" is uttered. PRD are 70% more likely to divorce than the general population, often reporting the disease as a contributing factor.[26] Parents of younger patients also describe difficulty in helping their children's teachers and classmates understand their illness.

PROBLEM THREE: Inability to diagnose the disease early, which could result in more successful treatment

Higher treatment success rates have been experienced in some exclusive trials in which people are diagnosed "very early" and treated aggressively.[27, 28] However, it is unlikely that the average patient in the US can receive such early treatment, chiefly due to diagnostic criteria that mostly emphasize conspicuous swelling in the hands.

Most PRD experience symptoms of the disease—not necessarily hand-related—for a long time prior to diagnosis. "Fifty-two percent of patients reported that they had RA symptoms for longer than a year prior to diagnosis. Twenty-two percent reported having symptoms for five or more years prior to diagnosis."[29] (See the chart below.) Lack of awareness about the disease in the general public and in medical professionals also contributes to late diagnosis. Female patients especially experience longer physician referral delays,[30] tend to ignore painful symptoms until usual activities are particularly disrupted, and may be less assertive in obtaining care for "arthritis."

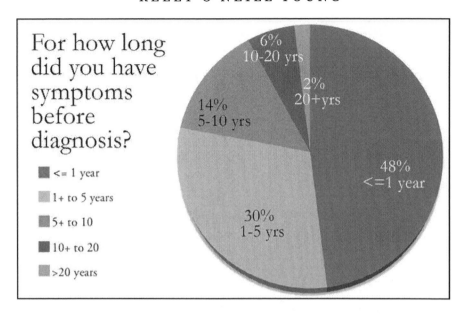

For how long did you have symptoms before diagnosis?

- ■ <= 1 year
- ■ 1+ to 5 years
- ■ 5+ to 10
- ■ 10+ to 20
- ■ >20 years

6% 10-20 yrs
2% 20+yrs
14% 5-10 yrs
48% <=1 year
30% 1-5 yrs

Inadequacies in the diagnostic process that contribute to the delay are related to reliance upon the conception of the disease as a "type of arthritis."[31] Doctors predominantly diagnose according to the visible appearance of the back of the hands because they were trained to think of RA as a "type of arthritis" which begins with conspicuous swelling of the MCP joints.[32, 33]

If followed strictly, the current diagnostic criteria make it virtually impossible to be diagnosed without conspicuous hand swelling.[34]

Typical media articles about RA mistakenly state that it begins with or merely involves inflammation of the small joints of the hands or feet.[35, 36, 37, 38, 39] The problem is that patients say any one of a dozen symptoms may occur as the first symptom of the disease (see Chapter 4). The disease may first become evident in the hands in some patients, but most report that it begins in other joints or with extra-articular symptoms.

What is needed is a systemic approach to diagnosis with a method of classification that is not dependent upon a single subjective variable symptom of the disease: conspicuous joint swelling in the hands.

The first step must be for clinicians and investigators to think beyond "arthritis," since there is evidence that the joint is not the site where the disease originates. Actual patient experiences in early disease[40] must be considered in order to improve diagnostic methods and measures for disease activity. Then it will be possible to educate general physicians and the public to identify early signs of the disease so it can be treated it earlier.

> "IT IS A DESTRUCTIVE SYSTEMIC DISEASE THAT
> AFFECTS ALL JOINTS IN THE BODY."
>
> HAMDAN ET AL.

(Footnote.)[41]

THE ARTHRITIS OF RD: SIMILARLY UNDERESTIMATED AND MISUNDERSTOOD

The balance of this book looks beyond the arthritis—joint inflammation—of RD. But questions related to that arthritis are also fraught with confusion. The following section addresses some common misconceptions.

Any joint can be affected by RD, and some PRD live with every joint affected. It's common to hear patients comment about problems in joints that they were not even aware of before RD affected them. Active disease often affects the cervical spine (neck), knees, shoulders, elbows, feet, hands, wrists, ankles, and rib-sternum joints. People with very active rheumatoid disease may also notice symptoms in the jaw, hip, vocal cord, sternoclavicular, thoracic, or lumbar spine joints.

Joint symptoms are often symmetrical, but not necessarily simultaneous. Joints on both sides will likely be involved, but symmetry does not require that both are similarly swollen or painful on the same day. Joint symptoms typically include the five signs of inflammation: swelling, redness, pain, stiffness, and warmth. However all five symptoms are not always present at the same time. Genetic variations account for differences in symptom presentation. And RD usually progresses over time, presenting differently over a period of years.

Extended periods of uncontrolled active disease can lead to bone erosion or to damage to connective tissues that leads to deformity. However, long before explicit deformity, inflammation of membranes around tendons and other connective tissues can be immediately disabling, even in very early disease. Before obvious deformity and permanent destruction, most patients experience what many call the "invisible" disability of RD. PRD often talk about feeling "frozen" or "rusty" because movement becomes very difficult, even impossible, at times. It is little acknowledged that the slow process toward discernible destruction or deformity is usually extremely painful and abruptly disabling. Many people, even doctors, are confused because they assume that pain and disability only result from eventual joint destruction when pain and disability are often caused by disease activity in connective tissue.

Disease modifying anti-rheumatic drugs (DMARDs) and biologic DMARDs generate a wide range of responses in the arthritis of RD. A minority of patients has a measurably good response in reduced joint symptoms, but one-third shows less than twenty percent improvement, or no response. The remainder, about 15 to 20%, experience moderate improvement (usually measured as about 50% reduced swelling).

These varying treatment response rates, along with variable

disease activity, sometimes called "flares," make it difficult to apprehend rheumatoid disease activity. RD can either exacerbate intermittently or progress steadily; however, even intermittently exacerbating joint symptoms can produce progressive changes and lead to damage. Rarely, PRD respond well enough to treatment to stop all joint symptoms or forestall disease progression.

Unfortunately, public information about the arthritis of RD incorrectly conveys that it is mostly limited to the hands or hands and feet and easily managed with modern medicine. Even medical professionals are frequently misinformed about the arthritis of RD: they are taught to look for MCP (metacarpophalangeal) joints with overt symmetrical swelling, redness, and warmth, although joints seldom appear in patients the way they are depicted in textbooks or on websites. A common misunderstanding of RD disability is that it occurs in late-stage disease as a result of bone destruction. And in the absence of bone erosion or obvious deformity, doctors sometimes suspect that joint pain is psychosomatic.

Most descriptions of rheumatoid arthritis seem milder and more easily managed than what PRD encounter. In the large online RA Warrior community, people have frequently expressed distress about problems caused by these inconsistencies. Discrepancy between patient and doctor estimation of disease activity is also very common.[42, 43, 44, 45] When misinformation about RD arthritis symptoms delays aggressive disease treatment, PRD are harmed because earlier treatment is known to be more effective.

One very straightforward example is synovitis and tenosynovitis: rheumatologists often tend to glance at the top (or back) of the hand looking for MCP synovitis. Meanwhile, PRD experience tenosynovitis that leads to deformity and causes pain, stiffness, and sudden disability especially in early disease.[46, 47, 48] Tendon-related inflammation, nodules, or damage would be more apparent on the palm side of the hand or might be detected with musculoskeletal ultrasound[49] (rarely used in the U.S.).

Sadly, even if the joint disease of RD were always recognized and measured appropriately, extra-articular (non-joint) symptoms are not measured, documented, or treated as part of disease activity levels. I hope that the evidence presented in this book will stimulate more such consideration.

Patients' perspectives on rheumatoid disease

In the next chapter, we will look at the dramatic history of the dangers of RD. The following passage, adapted from a 2012 article on rawarrior.com,[50] provides a glimpse into the evolution of my opinion about classifying RD as a type of arthritis.

WE REFUSE TO BE MISLABELED: UPDATING RHEUMATOID ARTHRITIS (RA)

Three years ago, I saw RA patients insisting that the name of the disease needed to be changed. They argued that until arthritis is removed from the name, confusion about the disease will continue. When asked, I said that we could not wait around for that to happen; let's work for awareness right now whatever the name is. And I did.

It seemed that changing the name of a disease is a decision that is not in the realm of patients. We can't do that. It's a job for organizations. With money. Who already control things. Which are not working well on behalf of patients... Hmm.

What changed my mind?

1) You did.

Spending 60 hours a week communicating with other people with rheumatoid disease converted me.

Without my encouragement, people continued to press the idea that a name change was necessary. Countless people told me that they see a name change as a key part of the awareness solution.

2) The facts convinced me.

The fact is that Rheumatoid is not a type of arthritis. Arthritis is one symptom of Rheumatoid Disease.

As I objectively studied the problem, I pulled apart threads like tangled yarn. Examining the origins of the confusion about rheumatoid disease leads to clear conclusions about what must be done to correct it. The word "arthritis" is one unambiguous thread. My learning process included writing over 800 articles for this site and various other publications.

3) An RA/RD foundation: the Rheumatoid Patient Foundation.

A few say we must first spend our energy convincing other organizations that they must change their ideals or goals to align with those of rheumatoid patients and give us what we need. Do people with other conditions or causes wait to be given whatever change they need? No, they demand it. A year ago, we created the Rheumatoid Patient Foundation, which *represents rheumatoid patients themselves.*

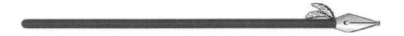

KEY POINTS

1. Remission is rare in the real world, but experts are accomplishing it with aggressive treatment in early disease.

2. Doctors measure by swelling, but swelling at a single moment does not represent the disease activity for the duration between appointments. Swelling does not correlate with damage. New research finds inflammation is separate from damage. Swelling is only one of many joint symptoms.

3. Which symptoms are RD?

RD is made up of

     a. Constitutional symptoms – like fever or fatigue

     b. Musculoskeletal disease – joints and connective tissues

     c. Extra-articular disease – organs and body systems affected by the disease

Not part of the RD

     a. Comorbidities – other illnesses and diagnoses

     b. Side effects – problems caused by medications

     c. Complications – other problems caused by treatment or surgery

4. Misunderstanding of the disease prevents early diagnosis.

5. Thinking of RD as arthritis interferes with research, relationships, work, and treatment.

Action step: The first step must be for clinicians and investigators to think beyond "arthritis," since there is evidence that the joint is not the site where the disease originates

Quote to remember: "When misinformation about RD arthritis symptoms delays aggressive disease treatment, PRD are harmed because earlier treatment is known to be more effective."

---

[1] Adams RF. An identity crisis for RA. (See footnote in Introduction.)

[2] Science Daily [website]. US study suggests that tofacitinib is an efficacious treatment for active rheumatoid arthritis. 2011 May 25 [cited 2013 Mar 23]. Available from: http://www.sciencedaily.com/ releases/2011/05/110525110145.htm

[3] Singh JA, Christensen R, Wells GA, Suarez-Almazor ME, Buchbinder R, Lopez-Olivo MA, Tanjong Ghogomu E, Tugwell P. Biologics for rheumatoid arthritis: An overview of Cochrane reviews (review). Minneapolis, MN: John Wiley and Sons, Ltd. 2009 [cited 2013 Mar 17](4) Art. No.: CD007848. Available from: http:// www.cochranejournalclub.com/biologics-for-rheumatoid-arthritis-clinical/pdf/CD007848_abstract.pdf DOI: 10.1002/14651858.CD007848.pub2

[4] Wolfe F. How am I doing? How are we doing? It all depends. National Databank for Rheumatic Diseases. 2011 Jan [cited 2013 Mar 17]. Available from: http://www.arthritis-research.org/participate/ newsletter/january-2011/how-am-i-doing-how-are-we-doing-it-all-depends

[5] Studenic P, Radner H, Smolen JS, Aletaha D. Discrepancies between patients and physicians in their perceptions of rheumatoid arthritis disease activity. Arthritis Rheum. 2012 Sep [cited 2013 Mar 23];64: 2814–2823. Available from: http://onlinelibrary.wiley.com/doi/10.1002/art.34543/full DOI: 10.1002/art.34543

[6] Rheumatoid Patient Foundation [website]. Unmasking rheumatoid disease: The patient experience of rheumatoid arthritis. A white paper from the Rheumatoid Patient Foundation. 2013 Apr 20 [cited 2013 Mar 28]. Available from: http://rheum4us.org/wp-content/uploads/2013/04/Unmasking-Rheumatoid-Disease-The-Patient-Experience-of-Rheumatoid-Arthritis-White-Paper.pdf

[7] Walsh N. MedPage Today Rheumatology [website]. 2016 Feb 10 [cited 2016 Feb 28]. Available from: http://www.medpagetoday.com/Rheumatology/Arthritis/56121

[8] Young K. Rheumatoid (arthritis) heart disease. Rheumatoid Arthritis Warrior [website]. 2011 Apr 27 [cited 2012 Sep 30]. Available from: http://rawarrior.com/rheumatoid-arthritis-heart-disease/

[9] Pappas D. Lung involvement. (See footnote in Chapter 1.)

[10] Jacobsson LT, Turesson C, Nilsson JA, Petersson IF, Lindqvist E, Saxne T, Geborek P. Treatment with TNF blockers and mortality risk in patients with rheumatoid arthritis. Ann Rheum Dis. 2007 May [cited 2013 Mar 23];66(5):670-675. Available from: http://www.ncbi.nlm.nih.gov/pmc/articles/PMC1954627/ DOI: 10.1136/ard.2006.062497

[11] Myasoedova E, Crowson CS, Matteson EL, Davis JM III, Therneau TM, Gabriel SE. Decreased cardiovascular mortality in patients with incident rheumatoid arthritis (RA) in recent years: Dawn of a new era in cardiovascular disease in RA? [abstract]. Arthritis Rheumatol. 2015 [cited 2017 Jun 18];67(suppl 10). Available from: http://

acrabstracts.org/abstract/decreased-cardiovascular-mortality-in-patients-with-incident-rheumatoid-arthritis-ra-in-recent-years-dawn-of-a-new-era-in-cardiovascular-disease-in-ra/

[12] Widdifield J, Paterson M, Huang A, Kuriya B, Thorne C, Pope JE, Bombardier C, Bernatsky S. Causes of death for patients with rheumatoid arthritis [abstract]. Arthritis Rheumatol. 2016 [cited 2017 Jun 17];68(suppl 10). Available from: http://acrabstracts.org/abstract/causes-of-death-for-patients-with-rheumatoid-arthritis/

[13] Jones C. Death by rheumatoid arthritis: Possible and preventable. Laurel, Md: Echelon Press LLC; 2010. 48 p.

[14] Na M-K, Chun H-J, Bak K-H, Yi H-J, Ryu JI, Han M-H. Risk factors for the development and progression of atlantoaxial subluxation in surgically treated rheumatoid arthritis patients, considering the time interval between rheumatoid arthritis diagnosis and surgery. Journal of Korean Neurosurgical Society. 2016 [cited 2017 Jun 18];59(6):590-596. DOI:10.3340/jkns.2016.59.6.590

[15] Massarotti EM, Solomon DH. The potential role of 'non-rheumatic' therapies in rheumatic disease. Arthritis Res Ther. 2013 Nov 6 [cited 2017 Jul 1];15:124. Available from: https://arthritis-research.biomedcentral.com/articles/10.1186/ar4371

[16] Yunt ZX, Solomon JJ. Lung disease in rheumatoid arthritis. Rheum Dis Clin North Am. 2015 May [cited 2017 Jul 9];41(2):225–236. Available from: https://www.ncbi.nlm.nih.gov/pmc/articles/PMC4415514/pdf/nihms-681678.pdf

[17] Arthritis Foundation [website]. Rheumatoid arthritis fact sheet. 2012 Mar 20 [cited 2013 Mar 13]. Available from: http://www.arthritis.org/files/images/AF_Connect/Departments/Public_Relations/Rheumatoid-Arthritis-Final-3-7-12.pdf

[18] Ellman P, Ball RE. Rheumatoid disease with joint and pulmonary manifestations. Brit Med J. 1948 Nov 6 [cited 2013 Apr 21];816-820.

Available From: http://www.ncbi.nlm.nih.gov/pmc/articles/
pmc2091941/pdf/brmedj03702-0014.pdf

[19] Barrett EM, Scott DG, Wiles NJ, Symmons DP. The impact of
rheumatoid arthritis on employment status in the early years of
disease: A UK community-based study. (Oxford) Rheumatology.
2000 Jul 24 [cited 2013 Mar 22];39 (12): 1403-1409. Available from:
http://rheumatology.oxfordjournals.org/content/39/12/1403.long

DOI: 10.1093/rheumatology/39.12.1403

[20] Allaire S, Wolfe F, Niu J, Lavalley MP. Contemporary prevalence
and incidence of work disability associated with rheumatoid arthritis
in the US. Arthrit Care Res. 2008 Apr 15 [cited 2013 Mar 22];59(4):
474-80. Available from: http://onlinelibrary.wiley.com/doi/
10.1002/art.23538/full DOI: 10.1002/art.23538

[21] Sokka T, Kautiainen H, Pincus T, Verstappen SM, Aggarwal A,
Alten R, Andersone D, Badsha H, Baecklund E, Belmonte M, et al.
Work disability remains a major problem in rheumatoid arthritis in
the 2000s: Data from 32 countries in the QUEST-RA study. Arthritis
Res Ther. 2010 [cited 2012 Jul 19];12(2):R42. Available from: http://
www.ncbi.nlm.nih.gov/pmc/articles/PMC2888189/ DOI: 10.1186/
ar2951

[22] Rheumatoid Arthritis Warrior Fan Page. Facebook [website]. 2013
Mar 18 [cited 2013 Mar 22]. Available from: http://
www.facebook.com/arthritiswarrior/posts/10151532739495726

[23] Young K. 5 Reasons disease awareness matters. Rheumatoid
Arthritis Warrior [website]. 2016 Feb 19 [cited 2017 Feb 24].
Available from: http://rawarrior.com/5-reasons-disease-awareness-
matters/

[24] Jamie, person with RA. In: Young K. RA can't be that bad – 5 Lies
and 5 replies. Rheumatoid Arthritis Warrior [website] 2017 Jun 9
[cited 2017 Jun 18]. Available from: http://rawarrior.com/ra-cant-

be-that-bad-5-lies-5-replies/?show=comments#comment-2433018

[25] Palmer KT, Brown I, Hobson, J, editors. Fitness for work: The medical aspects. 5th ed. Oxford (UK): Oxford University Press; 2013. p 282.

[26] Young K. Is rheumatoid arthritis a factor in divorce? Rheumatoid Arthritis Warrior [website]. 2012 May 29 [cited 2013 Mar 24]. Available from: http://rawarrior.com/is-rheumatoid-arthritis-a-factor-in-divorce/

[27] Gremese E, Salaffi F, Bosello SL, Ciapetti A, Bobbio-Pallavicini F, Caporali R, Ferraccioli G. Very early rheumatoid arthritis as a predictor of remission: A multicentre real life prospective study. Ann Rheum Dis. 2012 May 20 [cited 2013 Mar 24];0:1–5. Available from: http://ard.bmj.com/content/early/2012/07/12/ annrheumdis-2012-201456.full.pdf DOI: 10.1136/ annrheumdis-2012-201456

[28] Vermeer M, Kuper HH, Hoekstra M, Haagsma CJ, Posthumus MD, Brus HL, van Riel PL, van de Laar MA. Implementation of a treat-to-target strategy in very early rheumatoid arthritis: Results of the Dutch Rheumatoid Arthritis Monitoring remission induction cohort study. Arthritis Rheum. 2011 Oct [cited 2013 Mar 23];63(10): 2865-72. Available from: http://onlinelibrary.wiley.com/doi/ 10.1002/art.30494/full DOI: 10.1002/art.30494

[29] Rheumatoid Patient Foundation. Unmasking rheumatoid disease: The patient experience of rheumatoid arthritis. (See footnote Chapter 2.)

[30] Palm Ø, Purinszky E. Women with early rheumatoid arthritis are referred later than men. Ann Rheum Dis. 2005 [cited 2013 Mar 24]; 64:1227-1228. Available from: http://ard.bmj.com/content/ 64/8/1227.full.pdf DOI: 10.1136/ard.2004.031716

[31] Arthritis Foundation. Rheumatoid arthritis fact sheet. (See footnote

Chapter 2.)

[32] Maini RN, Venables PJW. Patient information: Rheumatoid arthritis symptoms and diagnosis (beyond the basics). UpToDate [website]; Wolters Kluwer Health. 2012 Mar 26 [cited 2013 Mar 30]. Available from: http://www.uptodate.com/contents/rheumatoid-arthritis-symptoms-and-diagnosis-beyond-the-basics

[33] Fields TR. Medical management of arthritis: Early diagnosis and current therapies. Hospital for Special Surgery [website]. 2005 Aug 2 [cited 2013 Mar 24]. Available from: http://www.hss.edu/professional-conditions_medical-management-arthritis-diagnosis-therapies.asp

[34] American College of Rheumatology; Atlanta (GA) [website]. The 2010 ACR-EULAR classification criteria for rheumatoid arthritis. 2010 Aug 10 [cited 2013 Mar 24]. Available from: http://www.rheumatology.org/practice/clinical/classification/ra/ra_2010.asp

[35] Dooren JC, Fox Business [website]. 2012 May 9 [cited 2013 May 4].

[36] Dooren JC. FDA panel recommends approval of Pfizer's tofacitinib. Advfn.com [website]. 2012 May [cited 2016 Mar 4]. Available from: http://www.advfn.com/nyse/StockNews.asp?stocknews=PFE&article=52346505

(Note: due to the previous webpages being no longer being available, this reference is provided as a similar concurrent reference.)

[37] Sturges M. Study shows vitamin D deficiency is related to diminished quality of life in rheumatoid arthritis patients. Vitamin D Council [website]. 2015 May 1 [cited 2017 Feb 24]. Available from: https://www.vitamindcouncil.org/study-shows-vitamin-d-deficiency-is-related-to-diminished-quality-of-life-in-rheumatoid-arthritis-patients/

38 Seetharaman M. Rheumatoid arthritis: In and out of the joint. Medscape [website]. 2017 Mar 16 [cited 2017 Jun 18]. Available from: http://reference.medscape.com/slideshow/rheumatoid-arthritis-6006748

39 Washington State University. Eureka Alert [website]. Compound in green tea found to block rheumatoid arthritis. 2016 Feb 16[cited 2017 Feb 24]. Available from https://www.eurekalert.org/pub_releases/2016-02/wsu-cig021616.php

40 Young K. Onset of rheumatoid arthritis stories. Rheumatoid Arthritis Warrior [website]. 2009 Oct 22 [cited 2016 Feb 28]. Available from: http://rawarrior.com/onset-of-rheumatoid-arthritis-stories/

41 Hamdan AL, Sarieddine D. Laryngeal manifestations of rheumatoid arthritis. Autoimmune Diseases. 2013 May 23 [cited 2017 Feb 26];2013. Article ID 103081. Available from: https://www.hindawi.com/journals/ad/2013/103081/

42 Studenic P, Radner H, Smolen JS, Aletaha D. Discrepancies between patients and physicians in their perceptions of rheumatoid arthritis disease activity. Arthritis Rheum. 2012 Aug 27 [cited 2017 Feb 25];64: 2814–2823. DOI: 10.1002/art.34543

43 Khan NA, Spencer HJ, Abda E, Aggarwal A, Alten R, Ancuta C, Andersone D, Bergman M, Craig-Muller J, Detert J, et al. Determinants of discordance in patients' and physicians' rating of rheumatoid arthritis disease activity. Arthritis Care Res. 2012 Feb [cited 2017 Feb 25];64(2):206-14. DOI: 10.1002/acr.20685.

44 Brown T. Patients rate RA disease activity worse than physicians do. Medscape [website]. 2012 Jul 19 [cited 2017 Feb 25]. Available from: http://www.medscape.com/viewarticle/767790

45 Young K. Disparity between rheumatoid arthritis patients & doctors over disease activity. RA Warrior [website]. 2012 Aug 3 [cited

2017 Feb 25]. Available from: http://rawarrior.com/disparity-between-rheumatoid-arthritis-patients-doctors-over-disease-activity/

[46] Nieuwenhuis WP, Krabben A, Stomp W, Huizinga TWJ, van der Heijde D, Bloem J L, van der Helm-van Mil A H M, Reijnierse M. Evaluation of magnetic resonance imaging–detected tenosynovitis in the hand and wrist in early arthritis. Arthritis Rheum. 2015 Mar 27 [cited 2017 Feb 25]; 67: 869–876. DOI:10.1002/art.39000

[47] Sahbudin I, Pickup L, Cader Z, Abishek A, Buckley CD, Allen G, Nightingale P, de Pablo P, Raza K, Filer A. Ultrasound-defined tenosynovitis is a strong predictor of early rheumatoid arthritis. Ann Rheum Dis. 2015 [cited 2017 Feb 25];74, Suppl 2. Available from: http://ard.bmj.com/content/74/Suppl_2/69.3

[48] Young K. Does rheumatoid arthritis affect tendons? RA Warrior [website]. 2013 Apr 12 [cited 2017 Feb 25]. Available from: http://rawarrior.com/does-rheumatoid-arthritis-affect-tendons/

[49] Bruyn GAW, Hanova P, Iagnocco A, Maria-Antonietta d'Agostino MA, Möller I, Terslev L, Backhaus M, Balint PV, Filippucci E, Baudoin P, et. al. on behalf of the OMERACT Ultrasound Task Force, et. al. Ultrasound definition of tendon damage in patients with rheumatoid arthritis. Results of a OMERACT consensus-based ultrasound score focussing on the diagnostic reliability, Ann Rheum Dis. 2014 Sep 16 [cited 2017 Feb 26];73:1929-1934. Available from: http://ard.bmj.com/content/73/11/1929

[50] Young, K. We refuse to be mislabeled. Rheumatoid Arthritis Warrior [website]. 2012 Jan 3 [cited 2013 Apr 27]. Available from: http://rawarrior.com/we-refuse-to-be-mislabeled-updating-rheumatoid-arthritis-ra-to-rheumatoid-autoimmune-disease-rad/

CHAPTER THREE
THE UNFOLDING STORY
OF RHEUMATOID DISEASE

Background for a disease perspective of rheumatoid disease

Prevalence of RD

It was a nameless disease for most of human history. Then some called it simply rheumatism. The disease was little discussed, but it was by no means rare. We have already covered some of the factors that contributed to the misconception that few people suffer from rheumatoid disease: patients suffered quietly, they went years before proper diagnosis, and few dollars were allocated for research. Many also live with the disease outside of the medical system because treatments are ineffective.

However, RA/RD is not a rare disease at all. Mayo Clinic says the lifetime risk of RA is 3.6 percent for women and 1.7 percent for men, with an overall risk of 2.4 percent. As a comparison, they mention that lifetime risk of all kinds of breast cancer for women is about 12 percent.[1] They calculate lifetime risk of all kinds of rheumatic inflammatory disease as 8.4 percent. See the chart below.

Disease	Women	Men
RA / RD	3.6% (1 in 28)	1.7 (1 in 59)
Polymyalgia rheumatica	2.4%	1.7
Lupus (SLE)	0.9%	0.2%
Giant cell arteritis	1.0%	0.5%
Psoriatic arthritis	0.5%	0.6%
Primary Sjogren's	0.8%	0.04%
Ankylosing spondylitis	0.1%	0.6%

There are wide variations in reports of the prevalence of RA, which seems to fluctuate unexpectedly.[2] Prevalence also seems to vary with various native populations. However, researchers agree that approximately one to three percent of the population has RA.[3, 4, 5, 6, 7, 8, 9, 10] The U.S. population is currently about 323 million, which would mean that there would be at least 3 million people in the U.S. with RA (or adjusted to count adults only, between 2.4 and 4.8 million). Hospital for Special Surgery in New York estimates that RA affects three million in the U.S.[11] Many of those people may remain in the shadows; popularly quoted estimates of those actually diagnosed and treated for RA in the U.S. range from 1.3 to 2.1 million.

Explanations for these inconsistencies include (1) the number of PRD in either early or late stage disease who do not pursue medical treatment due to perceptions of risks and benefits or previous lack of response to treatments; (2) people with preference for non-traditional treatments; and (3) people affected by the disease who are undiagnosed or misdiagnosed. A survey of patients found over half of PRD reported that they had RA symptoms for longer than a year prior to diagnosis, and over one in five reported RA symptoms for five or more years prior to diagnosis.[12]

History of rheumatoid disease

For at least four hundred years, the disease that we now recognize as RA has been observed and examined. By studying human remains, particularly Native Americans and Egyptians, some historians assert that the disease has existed for thousands of years. Progress in the development of treatments was non-existent through most of that time. In the twentieth century, science gradually identified and separated several other rheumatic diseases from the category of RA, such as gout and ankylosing spondylitis.

> "ELEVATED SCORES ON THE MMPI HYPOCHONDRIASIS, DEPRESSION, AND HYSTERIA SCALES
> RESULT FROM THEIR CHRONIC DISEASE
> RATHER THAN FROM PSYCHOLOGICAL ABNORMALITIES."
> 1986, PINCUS ET AL.

(Footnote.)[13]

The history of RD is filled with myths, confusion, and errors. From notions of a "rheumatoid personality"[14, 15] to suppositions that symptoms are caused by feminine bodily processes, to the insistence that it is a localized disease,[16] to assumptions that patients are embellishing symptoms,[17, 18] error has reigned. Such misunderstandings have stemmed from three historical facts:

1. Most RD symptoms are not visible to the naked eye

2. 75-80 percent of patients have been female while virtually all physicians were male

3. Objective testing methods verifying the presence of disease activity have been limited

Historically, no broadly effective treatments have existed. Patients relied on natural aspirin-like substances. In the twentieth century, patients used high doses of aspirin tablets for limited relief as well as hot mineral baths and assistive devices to cope with the pain and disability. In the 1950's, cortisone, the first corticosteroid, was hailed as the miracle drug for RA.[19] However side effects from high doses were serious and irreversible; patients died or were permanently scarred with heart, skin, liver, bone, or eye damage. These anti-inflammatory medicines all brought partial relief of symptoms, but did not address the progressive effects of the disease on joints, organs, or the general health of the patient. The mortality rate has remained largely unchanged[20] and today about three-fourths of PRD still survive on regular doses of anti-inflammatory and pain medications, in spite of modern treatments.[21, 22]

Recent advances in understanding RD

Recent decades have brought greater progress in the understanding of the disease process. With regard to joints, musculoskeletal ultrasound (MSUS) and magnetic resonance imaging (MRI) have confirmed that inflammation is present even when swelling is not externally perceptible to clinicians.[23, 24] Several investigations have disproven false notions of the disease as a psychiatric breakdown or malfunctioning of pain thresholds.[25, 26] And many studies have established a physical foundation for the disease, suggesting a genetic explanation exists for the high incidence of RA among certain populations such as females[27] or Native Americans.[28] Various environmental triggers of immunity to citrullinated proteins have also been observed, further demonstrating the material nature of the disease.

Recent work at the Karolinska Institute has demonstrated how anti-citrullinated protein antibodies (ACPA) can be responsible for pain[29] and damage[30] in rheumatoid disease in the absence of apparent inflammation or swelling. "Thus, our data highlight a potential role of ACPA in the type of joint pain that precedes development of RA and/or persists despite medical control of the disease activity."[31] *ACPAs induce pain in mice without evidence of inflammation or swelling.* These findings are highly significant because one of the most common points of discordance between rheumatologists and PRD seeking help is the experience of joint pain before or without obvious swelling.

Further, Wigerblad et al. were able to reverse the state of ACPA-induced increased pain, "pointing to a direct causal relationship between ACPA, CXCL1/2 and pain." It is a crucial step to recognize that disease activity (like ACPA production) within tissues is expressed in real disease symptoms (like pain). That disease activity is hidden from the naked eye, causing many to doubt patient claims of so-called "invisible" symptoms, delaying or precluding appropriate disease management.

Note also that I differ with Wigerblad et al. on the wording of "joint pain that precedes the development of RA" since, to me, the ACPAs and the joint pain would be evidence that the patient already has RA/RD. However, Karolinska is speaking in terms of current "clinical" criteria for diagnosis. This is further discussed in Chapter 4 in the section "Pre-clinical disease activity."

For decades, it has been known that ACPAs are highly specific to RD, but it was not acknowledged until recently that they could have any particular role in disease activity. I have even met rheumatologists who say, "They don't do anything." Fortunately, investigators are also exploring the roles of ACPA in various aspects of the disease.

For example, better mouse models of RD are being developed to improve research and ultimately create better treatments. One grant from the U.S. National Institutes of Health (NIH) seeks to create a more "RA-like disease" for research by making ACPA-positive mice.[32] Another broad-based published study explores the relationship of various ACPAs to a typical heart problem in RD, changes in the left ventricle. Investigators have found higher ACPA levels to be associated with higher left ventricular mass index (LVMI) in people with RD, "potentially implicating autoimmune targeting of citrullinated proteins in myocardial remodelling in RA."[33]

ACPAs have also been shown to be present within atherosclerotic plaque. Geraldino-Pardilla et al. studied people with RD, but no known cardiovascular disease (CVD). They found high levels of anti-citrullinated histone 2B antibodies (a type of ACPA) were strongly associated with coronary artery calcification (CAC), a measure of atherosclerosis. This suggests that some ACPAs may have a role in the heart disease of RD.[34]

We are poised for a quantum leap in the understanding of this disease. How quickly it will emerge will be impacted by two things:

> 1) The extent of the inclusion of the full patient experience in research[35, 36] in order to foster a more accurate perception of the disease;

> 2) Embracing a more global conception of the disease, no longer limiting the disease to only one of its

symptoms, "arthritis."

> "ARTHRITIS MAY BE ONLY ONE MANIFESTATION
> OF RHEUMATOID DISEASE"
>
> 1976, BRITISH MEDICAL JOURNAL

(Footnote.)[37]

Historical use of the term rheumatoid disease

Historically, *rheumatism* and *rheumatoid disease* have been used to refer to the same condition that later became referred to as "rheumatoid arthritis."[38, 39] Research articles may use the terms "rheumatoid disease" and "rheumatoid arthritis" interchangeably.[40, 41, 42, 43, 44] Community doctors[45] and government agencies (such as the CDC)[46] use both terms. The term *disease* is also often used when discussing specific aspects of rheumatoid disease.[47, 48, 49] *Rheumatoid disease* has been more broadly used by researchers and clinicians outside of the U.S.[50, 51, 52, 53]

In 1948, Ellman and Ball advocated the use of the label "rheumatoid disease" as preferable to "rheumatoid arthritis." They emphasized the many serious systemic manifestations that they had observed in patients, determining that the latter term misrepresented what they called the "rheumatoid state" which consists of "widespread pathological changes in various tissues and organs." Their conclusion: **From those observations, and in view of the widespread systemic nature of some of the cases, it will be understood how the term 'rheumatoid arthritis' is really misleading.** 'Rheumatoid disease' may be open to criticism, but it is preferable as the parent term, with joint lesions seen as the principal clinical manifestation, in the same way that the term 'gout' describes the parent lesions of a metabolic dysfunction whose principal clinical manifestation is the joint involvement."[54]

In 1963, Waine utilized the terms interchangeably:

"Next in feasibility is the arrest or moderation of rheumatoid disease in specific joints or other organs."[55]

And...

"The most desirable aim, but the least certain, is the defervescence of rheumatoid arthritis as a general disease of connective tissue."

Waine used "arthritis" to refer to joint symptoms; however, when discussing treatment, he favored "rheumatoid disease":

"When rheumatoid disease is diagnosed, the physician should make a most deliberate decision. Without first trying one or the other 'specific' drugs, will he accept responsibility of comprehensive management for an indefinite period? If so, he should define the patient's individual pattern and status in the variable course of rheumatoid disease. The goals for antirheumatic therapy must then be coordinated with the patient's personal and vocational needs. As the first step in management, the patient and often some members of the family, should be given a general orientation on the nature of the disease, the rationale of the basic program, the concept of control vs. cure, the need for active self-help, the limitations of drug therapy, and the essence of planned living."

In 1966, Conlon, et al. used the terms interchangeably, but also applied "rheumatoid disease" to joint degeneration of the spine: "These radiographs were subsequently read independently by two observers, with particular regard to the presence or absence of features previously suggested as common in or characteristic of rheumatoid disease and degenerative change."[56] Conlon and colleagues conducted the first large investigation to establish the frequency at which RD affects the cervical spine. They concluded that cervical spine involvement is so common that it should be used to help determine diagnosis of "definite rheumatoid arthritis." Their study of 333 patients found that cervical spine involvement correlated closely with peripheral destructive changes, but to a lesser degree with rheumatoid nodules and blood tests (rheumatoid factor).

Revelation of a systemic disease with many extra-articular features

In 1976, Fleming et al. studied "Extra-articular features in early rheumatoid disease," crediting Bauer and Clark (1948) with advancing the model of a systemic approach to rheumatoid disease.[57] Fleming's team found arthritis to be only one "manifestation of rheumatoid disease." Because there existed "little information on the occurrence of extra-articular features within the first few years" of the disease, they conducted a 4.5-year trial with 102 PRD who presented within the first year of onset.

Fleming's study demonstrated the trait of every great researcher or clinician, too often absent with current assumptions about "rheumatoid arthritis": *intellectual curiosity*. The study's methods were comparable to what is presently referred to as "patient reported outcome measures." Fleming's team systematically documented clinical examinations, interviews, laboratory results, and demographic data, acknowledging the unique value of the comprehensive data obtained through such methodology. Their findings:

> 1. High early incidence of extra-articular features in rheumatoid disease with 94 out of 102 patients showing

manifestations in the 4.5 years from disease onset

2. Only 8% showed no systemic manifestations and 41% had four or more

3. No significant associations with age, the presence of rheumatoid factor, or radiological erosions

4. Percentage showing positive rheumatoid factor increased from 40% to 66% during trial period

5. Being underweight early in the disease heralds a more severe form of the disease

6. While many features were only clinically detectable intermittently, most PRD tended toward decline, with a milder outcome evident in others: Overall 26 patients improved, 14 pursued a mild steady course, and 62 pursued a persistently severe or deteriorating course.

Note that in 1976 cardiovascular disease was not yet widely considered as a direct complication or manifestation of RD, and incidences of CV involvement were not obvious by the methods of investigation used in this trial. However, the authors noted that one patient who died suddenly (not being identified as having had cardiovascular involvement) was shown by autopsy to have "gross rheumatoid cardiac involvement at necropsy with multiple nodules in the myocardium and rupture through a softened nodule near the sinus of Valsalva." (For more on cardiovascular rheumatoid disease, see Chapter 5.)

Even without the technologically advanced tools we have today, *this study disproved certain misconceptions such as the common belief that extra-articular manifestations occur as features of later stage disease.* My experience with patients and several research studies cited in this book show that this common notion is wrong. According to Yunt and Solomon, "Mortality in RA is greatest within the first 5 to 7 years after diagnosis," and RD lung disease accounts for 10 to 20 percent of those deaths.[58]

Careful study prompted Fleming, et al. to conclude that they should title that article, and some subsequent works, with the term *rheumatoid disease*. One value of Fleming's research is that it demonstrates the power of preconceptions. Being conscious that one is investigating or treating a "disease" provokes more complex observations than are likely with a "type of arthritis." Researchers use more elaborate methods of investigation and ask different questions.

Preconceptions of clinicians, in part, account for the discrepancy between patient and clinician-based reports concerning the incidence of extra-articular manifestations of rheumatoid disease.[59] This can also account for the correlation between patient reports of particular manifestations and autopsy studies.

"RHEUMATOID DISEASE (RD) IS A COMMON CHRONIC INFLAMMATORY CONDITION ASSOCIATED WITH PROGRESSIVE JOINT DESTRUCTION. SUFFERERS OF RD EXPERIENCE REDUCED LIFE EXPECTANCY, REFLECTED IN THE INCREASED STANDARISED MORTALITY RATES REPORTED IN SEVERAL STUDIES OVER THE LAST 50 YEARS. MOST STUDIES INDICATE THAT THE INCREASED MORTALITY AFFECTING THIS POPULATION IS MAINLY DUE TO CARDIO-VASCULAR DISEASE."
2006, JOURNAL OF THE AMERICAN COLLEGE OF CARDIOLOGY

(Footnote.)[60]

Mortality in rheumatoid disease

Researchers have identified an increased risk of mortality from

RD, but have been unable to say what will change that. People with RD have a significantly increased risk of death compared with age- and sex-matched controls without RD from the same community. "The determinants of this excess mortality remain unclear; however, reports suggest increased risk from gastrointestinal, respiratory, cardiovascular, infectious, and hematologic diseases among RA patients compared with controls."[61] Unlike many conditions, no one can tell people how to avoid developing RD or decrease their risk of death.

One of the facts that has been confirmed over the past decade of research is the higher incidence of cardiovascular deaths compared with the general population.[62] While little is known about why, the mortality gap has widened for people with rheumatoid disease.[63] Lifespan is estimated to be shortened by five to fifteen years. Some reports show mortality for PRD is not improving overall,[64, 65, 66, 67] while others show mortality improvement with substantial disparities between populations.[68] In a session at the 2016 annual meeting of the American College of Rheumatology in Washington, D.C., Dr. Sherine Gabriel, a pioneer in research of mortality and cardiovascular disease in RD and dean of the Robert Wood Johnson Medical School, also reported such disparities in mortality improvement.[69]

However, accurate statistics with regard to RD mortality are difficult to obtain.[70] Numerous studies have also recognized serious underreporting of RA on death certificates[71, 72, 73, 74, 75, 76, 77, 78] and that generally, "autoimmune diseases tend to be underreported on death certificates."[79]

Not only do death certificates of PRD often fail to reflect their RA status, but usually death certificates of PRD also fail to mention extra-articular disease and other specific disease information that could have had bearing on determining cause of death.[80, 81] Although the disease is likely to be an underlying reason for the immediate cause of death, the disease itself is usually not cited on death certificates.[82, 83] One study demonstrated that physicians underreport RA as related to cause of death.[84] Another difficulty is that systemic effects of RD, such as rheumatoid heart disease or amyloidosis, are often undetected or considered asymptomatic.[85, 86] This is so, despite the fact that worse disease portends higher mortality risk.[87, 88, 89]

The label of RA as "a type of arthritis" could be at least partially responsible for such widespread error in death record management.

Molina et al. investigated factors associated with recording RA on death certificates.[90] They found younger PRD and those with more obvious joint deformities and fewer "comorbidities" were more likely to have RA accurately reported on their death certificates. Several patients diagnosed with overlapping musculoskeletal conditions to RA such as Sjögren's syndrome, Raynaud's phenomenon, or SLE (systemic lupus erythematosus), had that other condition mentioned, but not RA.

The results demonstrate a striking contrast to patients with SLE: 60% of the time, SLE was correctly mentioned on death certificates, while RA was only accurately recorded 19.5% of the time. Obviously, these other rheumatic diseases (SLE, Raynaud's, etc.) do not have "arthritis" attached to their names. This suggests that officials signing death certificates might be affected by the apparent triviality implied by the word arthritis, and consequently be misled that RA would not be as relevant to record as SLE or Sjögren's.

Molina et al. also note that the problem of death certificates for PRD has seen no progress in 30 years since it was first documented. This may have an effect on epidemiological research: "Therefore, incomplete or inaccurate records have many implications for research that rely on these records. Given that diseases of the musculoskeletal system are not often considered immediate causes of death, completeness of recording underlying conditions in the death certificate becomes crucial when analyzing mortality of these diseases."[91]

> "WITHOUT IDENTIFYING RA AS AN UNDERLYING CONDITION, EPIDEMIOLOGICAL STUDIES THAT RELY ON INFORMATION FROM DEATH CERTIFICATES MAY NOT FULLY ASCERTAIN THE MORBIDITY AND MORTALITY OF THE DISEASE."
>
> 2015, MOLINA ET AL.

(Footnote.)[92]

Do we know how many people are affected by rheumatoid disease?

The following passage is adapted from an article on rawarrrior.com[93]

HOW MANY PEOPLE HAVE RHEUMATOID ARTHRITIS?

The old adage seems apt: Statistics means never having to say you're certain.

Do we know conclusively how many people actually have RA? How many are being treated for "Rheumatoid Arthritis" in the U.S.? Or how likely a person is to be diagnosed with it in his or her lifetime?

Not really.

Apparently, it's a bit slippery.

In 2009, Gabriel and Michaud observed "a recent systematic review of the incidence and prevalence of RA revealed substantial variation in incidence and prevalence across the various studies and across time periods within the studies."[94] In that study, they reported a suspected decline in the incidence of RA. However, a year later, Mayo Clinic reported that fifty years of data showed the incidence of RA in the U.S. was actually climbing.[95] Publications from Mayo Clinic have estimated between 1.6 and 2.1 million U.S cases in recent years. They also found the lifetime risk of RA to be 3.6 percent for women and 1.7 percent for men.

The Centers for Disease Control and Prevention (CDC) lists RA on its "arthritis" page of its data section. According to CDC, an estimated 1.5 million adults had rheumatoid arthritis in 2007.[96] The American College of Rheumatology regularly estimates the number of Americans with RA at 1.3 million.[97]

One arthritis organization consistently says "more than a million" in the U.S. have RA.[98]

How can we know what's accurate?

1) Use genetics?

23andMe (a direct-to-consumer genetic testing company) estimates genetic risk for many diagnoses, including RA. Their website says, "2.4 out of 100 men of European ethnicity will get Rheumatoid Arthritis between the ages of 18 and 79," estimating the genetic risk of RA to be 2.4% for men and 4.2% for women (of European ancestry).[99] That's easy to remember. But genetic risk is only half of the story. Literally.

Researchers hypothesize that environmental triggers account for about 50% of the risk of developing RA. So we might expect only those with the genetic risk who are also exposed to certain triggers to actually develop the disease. This also lends logical explanation for the variance in incidence across time periods.

2) Work backwards?

According to the World Heath Organization (WHO), "the prevalence of definite or classical RA by the 1958 ARA or 1987 ACR criteria is approximately 1%."[100] This is a significant statement since those older diagnostic criteria allow for diagnosis of more advanced disease, which means fewer people were diagnosed. How many people are in the U.S.? 323,325,253 —according to the constantly updated U.S. Census Bureau's Population Clock. One percent of roughly 320 million is over 3 million.

3) Count them all?

Raise your hand high so we can see you in the back. Ouch. *Maybe not.*

It's obviously not feasible to count everyone with RD, but even extrapolating from a smaller population is problematic. Many people would not be counted because...

> a) People often have symptoms for a long time before being diagnosed with RA.
>
> b) Many give up and quit seeing rheumatologists or taking treatments.
>
> c) For a complete statistical picture, we need to include those diagnosed in childhood. About 300,000 people estimated to have juvenile RA in the U.S. are not counted as diagnosed with RA. But adults diagnosed

with RA commonly report symptoms extending back into childhood.

Statistics: a tool to correct misconceptions?

I read a remarkable article on stats this week, in terms of basketball.[101] "...Stats are here to stay. Showing up without them is like a carpenter showing up to work without a hammer. But statistics are a tool, not the tool. The carpenter needs a hammer, but you can't just go around hammering everything and calling it good."

Statistics are not the only tool, but an important tool. We need a better grip on this tool to help the millions of people living with RD. Correcting misconceptions about RD may be a good place to start.

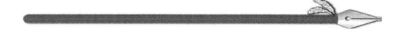

KEY POINTS

1. RD is not rare. It affects 1% of the population or about 2 and a half million adults in the U.S. RA occurs about 4 times as often as lupus.

2. Recent advances show disease activity directly causes pain and destruction, apart from swelling. Several myths and accusations about PRD have been proven false.

3. Rheumatoid disease is a historically advocated term still used in research.

4. Extra-articular disease occurs frequently and early on in RD.

5. It is difficult to study the higher mortality of RD because of severely low reporting on death certificates (only 19% reported).

6. Technology such as MRI and MSUS has helped to document disease activity even in the absence of obvious swelling.

Action step: Clinicians should recognize the many extra-articular effects of RD. And as science catches up with the reality of RD, they should trust that patients' symptoms are the result of disease activity, not depression or another scapegoat.

Quote to remember: "From those observations, and in view of the widespread systemic nature of some of the cases, it will be understood how the term 'rheumatoid arthritis' is really misleading." (See footnote Chapter 1, Ellman, Rheumatoid disease, 1948.)

---

[1] Mayo Clinic News [website]. Mayo clinic determines lifetime risk of adult rheumatoid arthritis. 2011 Jan 5 [cited 2013 Mar 23]. Available from: http://www.mayoclinic.org/news2011-rst/6137.html?rss-feedid=1

[2] Myasoedova E, Crowson CS, Kremers HM, Therneau TM, Gabriel SE. Is the incidence of rheumatoid arthritis rising? Results from Olmsted County, Minnesota, 1955-2007. Arthritis Rheum. 2010 [cited 2012 Sep 30];62(6):1576–1582. Available from: http://onlinelibrary.wiley.com/doi/10.1002/art.27425/full DOI: 10.1002/art.27425

[3] Bingham C, Ruffing V. Rheumatoid arthritis signs and symptoms. The Johns Hopkins Arthritis Center [website]. 2012 Nov 28 [cited 2012 Sep 30]. Available from: http://www.hopkinsarthritis.org/

arthritis-info/rheumatoid-arthritis/ra-symptoms/

[4] Australian Institute of Health and Welfare [website]. A snapshot of rheumatoid arthritis. 2013 May [cited 2017 Feb 26]. ISBN 978-1-74249-426-5. Available from: http://www.aihw.gov.au/WorkArea/DownloadAsset.aspx?id=60129543377

[5] Hamdan et al. Laryngeal manifestations of rheumatoid arthritis. (See footnote Chapter 2.)

[6] van Steenbergen HW, Huizinga, TWJ, van der Helm-van Mil AHM. Review: The preclinical phase of rheumatoid arthritis: What is acknowledged and what needs to be assessed? Arthritis Rheum. 2013 Sep [cited 2017 Mar4];65(9):2219–2232. DOI:10.1002/art.38013

[7] Cojocaru M, Cojocaru IM, Silosi I, Vrabie CD, Tanasescub R. Extra-articular manifestations in rheumatoid arthritis. Maedica (Buchar). 2010 Dec [cited 2017 Mar 4];5(4):286–291. Available from: https://www.ncbi.nlm.nih.gov/pmc/articles/PMC3152850/

[8] Molina E, del Rincon I, Restrepo JF, Battafarano DF, Escalante A. Mortality in rheumatoid arthritis (RA): Factors associated with recording RA on death certificates. BMC Musculoskeletal Disorders. 2015 Oct 5[cited 2017 Mar 5]16:277. DOI: 10.1186/s12891-015-0727-7

[9] Young K. How many people have rheumatoid arthritis? Rheumatoid Arthritis Warrior [website]. 2013 Mar 13 [cited 2013 Mar 23]. Available from: http://rawarrior.com/how-many-people-have-rheumatoid-arthritis/

[10] Lawrence RC, Helmick CG, Arnett FC, Deyo RA, Felson DT, Giannini EH, Heyse SP, Hirsch R, Hochherg MC, Hundek GG, et al. Estimates of the prevalence of arthritis and selected musculoskeletal disorders in the United States. Arthritis Rheum. 1998 May [cited 2016 Mar 5];41(5):778-799.

[11] Hospital for Special Surgery. [Press Release]. Hospital for Special Surgery receives grant for new genomics center to study autoimmune diseases. 2013 Apr 25 [cited 2013 May 4]. Available from: http://www.hss.edu/newsroom_genomics-center-study-autoimmune-diseases.asp

[12] Rheumatoid Patient Foundation. Unmasking rheumatoid disease. (See footnote Chapter 2.)

[13] Pincus et al. Elevated MMPI scores reflect disease. (See footnote in Chapter 1.)

[14] Arthritis Foundation. Good living with rheumatoid. (See footnote in Chapter 1.)

[15] Solomon GF, Moos RH. The relationship of personality to the presence of rheumatoid factor in asymptomatic relatives of patients with rheumatoid arthritis. Psychosom Med. 1965 [cited 2013 Mar 24];27(4):350-360. Available from: http://www.psychosomaticmedicine.org/content/27/4/350.full.pdf

[16] Bywaters EGL. Brief notes on the natural history of rheumatoid arthritis. Can Med Assoc J. 1964 Sep 12 [cited 2012 Sep 30]; 91:606-608. Available from: http://www.ncbi.nlm.nih.gov/pmc/articles/PMC1927420/pdf/canmedaj01065-0035.pdf

[17] Young K. Rheumatoid arthritis pain in the twilight zone. Rheumatoid Arthritis Warrior [website]. 2010 Feb 10 [cited 2012 Sep 30]. Available from: http://rawarrior.com/rheumatoid-arthritis-pain-in-the-twilight-zone/

[18] Young K. Does rheumatoid arthritis pain really hurt that much? Rheumatoid Arthritis Warrior [website]. 2010 Feb 18 [cited 2012 Sep 30]. Available from: http://rawarrior.com/does-rheumatoid-arthritis-pain-really-hurt-that-much/

[19] Mayo Clinic [website]. Nobel Prize Telegram. 2015 Jul 7 [cited 2016

Feb 28]. Available from: http://history.mayoclinic.org/historic-highlights/nobel-prize-telegram.php

[20] Gabriel SE. Why do people with rheumatoid arthritis still die prematurely? (See footnote in Chapter 1.)

[21] Strand V, Emery P, Fleming S, Griffin C. The impact of rheumatoid arthritis (RA) on women: Focus on pain, productivity and relationships [abstract]. Arthritis Rheum. 2010 [cited 2013 Mar 24]; 62 Suppl 10:1063. Available from: http://www.blackwellpublishing.com/acrmeeting/abstract.asp?MeetingID=774&id=89712 DOI: 10.1002/art.288302012

[22] Rheumatoid Patient Foundation. Unmasking rheumatoid disease. (See Footnote Chapter 2.)

[23] Brown AK, Quinn MA, Karim Z, Conaghan PG, Peterfy CG, Hensor E, Wakefield RJ, O'Connor PJ, Emery P. Presence of significant synovitis in rheumatoid arthritis patients with disease-modifying antirheumatic drug–induced clinical remission: Evidence from an imaging study may explain structural progression. Arthritis Rheum. 2006 Dec [cited 2013 Mar 24];54(12):3761–3773. Available from: http://onlinelibrary.wiley.com/doi/10.1002/art.22190/pdf DOI: 10.1002/art.22190

[24] Zoler ML. Ultrasound speeds new RA diagnoses. Rheumatology News [website]. 2013 Jul 11 [cited 2013 Aug 3]. Available from: http://www.rheumatologynews.com/specialty-focus/rheumatoid-arthritis/single-article-page/ultrasound-speeds-new-ra-diagnoses/

[25] O'Driscoll SL, Jayson MIV. The clinical significance of pain threshold measurements [abstract]. (Oxford) Rheumatology. 1982 [cited 2012 Sep 30];21(1):31-35. Available from: http://rheumatology.oxfordjournals.org/content/21/1/31.abstract DOI: 10.1093/rheumatology/21.1.31

[26] Pincus. Elevated MMPI scores reflect disease. (See footnote

Chapter 1.)

[27] Kvien TK, Uhlig T, Ødegård, S, Heiberg MS. Epidemiological aspects of rheumatoid arthritis: The sex ratio. Annals of the New York Academy of Sciences. 2006 Jun 30 [cited 2017 Jul 16]1069: 212–222. DOI: 10.1196/annals.1351.019

[28] Ferucci ED, Templin DW, Lanier AP. Rheumatoid arthritis in American Indians and Alaska natives: A review of the literature. Semin Arthritis Rheum. 2005 Feb [cited 2017 Jul 16];34(4):662-667. Available from: https://doi.org/10.1016/j.semarthrit.2004.08.003

[29] Wigerblad G, Bas DB, Fernades-Cerqueira C, Krishnamurthy A, Nandakumar KS, Rogoz K, Kato J, Sandor K, Su J, Jimenez-Andrade JM, et al. Autoantibodies to citrullinated proteins induce joint pain independent of inflammation via a chemokine-dependent mechanism. Ann Rheum Dis. 27 Nov 2016 [cited 2017 Mar 24]; 75:730–738. DOI: 10.1136/annrheumdis-2015-208094

[30] Krishnamurthy A, Joshua V, Hensvold AH, Jin T, Sun M, Vivar N, Ytterberg AJ, Engström M, Fernandes-Cerqueira C, Amara K, et al. Identification of a novel chemokine-dependent molecular mechanism underlying rheumatoid arthritis-associated autoantibody-mediated bone loss. Ann Rheum Dis. 2016 Apr 1 [cited 2017 Mar 24];75:721-729. Available from: http://ard.bmj.com/content/75/4/721

[31] Wigerblad G, et al. Autoantibodies to citrullinated proteins induce joint pain. (See footnote Chapter 3.)

[32] National Institutes of Health [website]. NIH research grant 5R03AR061593-03 displayed in Estimates of Funding for Various Research, Condition, and Disease Categories. 2017 Jul 2 [cited 2017 Aug 1] Available from: https://report.nih.gov/categorical_spending.aspx

[33] Geraldino-Pardilla L, Russo C, Sokolove J, Robinson WH, Zartoshti

A, Van Eyk J, Fert-Bober J, Lima j, Giles JT, Bathon JM. Association of anti-citrullinated protein or peptide antibodies with left ventricular structure and function in rheumatoid arthritis. (Oxford) Rheumatology. 2017 Apr 1 [cited 2017 Jul 3]56(4):534–540. DOI: 10.1093/rheumatology/kew436

34 Geraldino-Pardilla L, Giles JT, Sokolove J, Zartoshti A, Robinson WH, Budoff M, Detrano R, Bokhari S, Bathon JM. Association of anti–citrullinated peptide antibodies with coronary artery calcification in rheumatoid arthritis. Arthrit Care Res. 2017 Jul 10 [cited Jul 25];69(8):1276–1281. DOI:10.1002/acr.23106

35 Beal AC, Sheridan S. Matchmaker, matchmaker – The PCORI challenge initiative. Patient-Centered Outcomes Research Institute [website]. 2012 Dec 14 [cited 2013 Mar 24]. Available from: http://www.pcori.org/blog/matchmaker-matchmaker-the-pcori-challenge-initiative/

36 Pulse International: Fortnightly Medical Newspaper published from Pakistan [Internet]. Rheumatology Conference Proceedings-II. 2012 Nov 15 [cited 2013 Apr 27]. Available from: http://www.pulsepakistan.com/index.php/main-news-nov-15-12/119-early-use-of-dmards-can-prevent-disability-from-rheumatic-diseases-dr-mahboobur-rehman

37 Fleming A, Dodman S, et al. Extra-articular features in early rheumatoid disease. (See footnote in Chapter 1.)

38 Fleming A, Crown JM, Corbett M. Early rheumatoid disease. Ann Rheum Dis. 1976 [cited 2012 Jul 19];(35)357. Available from: http://www.ncbi.nlm.nih.gov/pmc/articles/PMC1007396/pdf/annrheumd00035-0070.pdf

39 Fleming A, Dodman S, et al. Extra-articular features in early rheumatoid disease. (See footnote in Chapter 1.)

40 Murphy TM. Surgical considerations of rheumatoid disease

involving the craniocervical junction and atlantoaxial vertebrae. In: Lemmey A, editor. Rheumatoid arthritis — etiology, consequences and co-Morbidities. Dublin (IL): InTech; 2012 Jan [cited 2012 Jul 19];275-304. Available from: http://cdn.intechweb.org/pdfs/ 25408.pdf

[41] Wells AU and Hirani N. Interstitial lung disease guideline. Thorax. 2008 [cited 2013 Jun 21];63:v1-v58. Available from: http:// thorax.bmj.com/content/63/Suppl_5/v1.full

[42] Goldfarb CA, Stern PJ. Metacarpophalangeal joint arthroplasty in rheumatoid arthritis, a long-term assessment. J Bone Joint Surg Am. 2003 Oct; 85[cited 2017 Feb 26];10:1869 -1878. Available from: http://jbjs.org/content/85/10/1869

[43] Kumar N, Armstrong DJ. Cardiovascular disease – The silent killer in rheumatoid arthritis. Clin Med. 2008 Aug [cited 2017 Mar 22]; 8(4):384–7. Available from: http://www.clinmed.rcpjournal.org/ content/8/4/384.full.pdf

[44] Friedman RJ, Thornhill TS, Thomas WH, Sledge CB. Non-constrained total shoulder replacement in patients who have rheumatoid arthritis and class-IV function. J Bone Joint Surg Am. 1989 Apr [cited 2017 Feb 26];71(4):494 -498. Available from: http:// jbjs.org/content/71/4/494

[45] Ibrahim M. Hand and wrist problems: Rheumatoid disease & the hand. Chicago (IL): American Society for Surgery of the Hand; Valley Hand Surgery [website]; 2009 [cited 2012 July 19]. Available from: http://www.stanmedplaza.com/ibrahim/rheumatoid.html

[46] Kotton CN, Freedman DO. Immunocompromised travelers. Centers for Disease Control and Prevention [website]. 2015 Sep 4 [cited 2016 Mar 5]. Available from: http://wwwnc.cdc.gov/travel/ yellowbook/2016/advising-travelers-with-specific-needs/ immunocompromised-travelers

[47] Wikipedia contributors. Rheumatoid lung disease. Wikipedia, The Free Encyclopedia [Internet]. c 2010-2013 [cited 2012 July 19]. Available from: http://en.wikipedia.org/wiki/Rheumatoid_lung_disease

[48] New York Times [website]. Rheumatoid lung disease. 2011 Jun 10 [cited 2012 Jul 19]. Available from: http://health.nytimes.com/health/guides/disease/rheumatoid-lung-disease/overview.html

[49] Harper SL, Foster CS. The ocular manifestations of rheumatoid disease. Int Ophthalmol Clin. 1998 Winter [cited 2012 Jul 19];38(1): 1-19. Available from: http://www.ncbi.nlm.nih.gov/pubmed/9532469

[50] Helmy M, Shohayeb M, Helmy MH, el-Bassiouni EA. Antioxidants as adjuvant therapy in rheumatoid disease. A preliminary study. Arzneimittelforschung. 2001 [cited 2012 July 19]; 51(4): 293-298. Available from: http://www.ncbi.nlm.nih.gov/pubmed/11367869 DOI: 10.1055/s-0031-1300040

[51] Bhatia GS, Sosin MD, Grindulis KA, Davis RC, Lip GY. Rheumatoid disease and the heart: From epidemiology to echocardiography. Expert Opin Investig Drugs. 2005 Jan [cited 2013 Apr 20];14(1): 65-76. DOI:10.1517/13543784.14.1.65)

[52] McGuigan L, Burke D, Fleming A. Tarsal tunnel syndrome and peripheral neuropathy in rheumatoid disease. Ann Rheum Dis. 1983 [cited 2013 Apr 20];42:128-131. Available from: http://ard.bmj.com/content/42/2/128.full.pdf

[53] Brewerton DA. Hand deformities in rheumatoid disease. Ann Rheum Dis. 1957 Feb 1 [cited 2017 Feb 26];)16,183. Available from: https://www.ncbi.nlm.nih.gov/pmc/articles/PMC1006945/pdf/annrheumd00181-0025.pdf

[54] Ellman P. Rheumatoid disease. (See footnote Chapter 2.)

[55] Waine H, Montgomery MM, Ensign DC. Management of the rheumatoid patient. Arthritis Rheum. 1963 Feb [cited 2013 Apr 27]; 6: 83–92. DOI: 10.1002/art.1780060111

[56] Conlon PW, Isdale IC, Rose BS. Rheumatoid arthritis of the cervical spine: An analysis of 333 cases. Ann Rheum Dis. 1966 [cited 2017 Jul 1];25:120-126. http://www.ncbi.nlm.nih.gov/pmc/articles/PMC2453383/pdf/annrheumd00507-0014.pdf

[57] Fleming A, Dodman S, et al. Extra-articular features in early rheumatoid disease. (See footnote in Chapter 1.)

[58] Yunt ZX. Lung disease in rheumatoid arthritis. (See footnote Chapter 2.)

[59] Rheumatoid Patient Foundation. Unmasking Rheumatoid Disease. (See footnote Chapter 2.)

[60] Bhatia GS, Sosin MD, Patel JV, Grindulis KA, Khattak FH, Hughes EA, Lip GYH, Davis RC. Left ventricular systolic dysfunction in rheumatoid disease : An unrecognized burden? J Am Coll Cardiol. 2006 Mar 21 [cited 2013 Apr 21];47(6): 1169–1174.

[61] Gabriel SE. The epidemiology of rheumatoid arthritis [abstract]. Rheum Dis Clin N Am. 2001 May [cited 2012 July 20];27(2):269-81. Available from: http://www.ncbi.nlm.nih.gov/pubmed/11396092001

[62] Meune C, Touzé E, Trinquart L, Allanore Y. Trends in cardiovascular mortality in patients with rheumatoid arthritis over 50 years: A systematic review and meta-analysis of cohort studies. (Oxford) Rheumatology. 2009 Aug [cited 2012 Jul 19];48(10): 1309-1313. Available from: http://rheumatology.oxfordjournals.org/content/48/10/1309.full DOI:10.1093/rheumatology/kep252

[63] Gonzalez A, Icen M, D, Kremers HM, Crowson CS, Davis JM, Therneau TM, Roger VL, Gabriel SE. Mortality trends in rheumatoid arthritis: The role of rheumatoid factor. J Rheumatol. 2008 Jun

[cited 2012 Jul 20];35(6):1009–1014. Available from: http://www.ncbi.nlm.nih.gov/pmc/articles/PMC2834198/

[64] Gabriel SE, Crowson CS, O'Fallon WM. Mortality in rheumatoid arthritis: Have we made an impact in 4 decades? [abstract]. J Rheumatol. 1999 Dec [cited 2016 Mar 5];26(12):2529-2533. Available from: http://www.ncbi.nlm.nih.gov/pubmed/10606358?dopt=Abstract

[65] Humphreys JH, Warner A, Chipping J, Marshall T, Lunt M, Symmons DPM, Verstappen SMM. Mortality trends in patients with early rheumatoid arthritis over 20 years: Results from the Norfolk Arthritis Register. Arthrit Care Res. 2014 Dec 27 [cited 2017 Jul 8]; 66:1296–1301. DOI:10.1002/acr.22296

[66] Boers M, Jijkmans B, Gabriel S, Maradit-Kremers H, O'Dell J, Pincus T. Making an impact on mortality in rheumatoid arthritis. Arthritis Rheum. 2004 [cited 2017 Feb 26];50:1734-9. Available from: http://onlinelibrary.wiley.com/doi/10.1002/art.20306/full

[67] Kvien TK. Epidemiology and burden of illness of rheumatoid arthritis. PharmacoEconomics. 2004 Sep [cited 2017 Jul 16]22(1);1–12. Available from: https://link.springer.com/article/10.2165/00019053-200422001-00002

[68] Kiadaliri AA, Felson DT, Neogi T, Englund M. Rheumatoid arthritis as underlying cause of death in 31 countries, 1987-2011: Trend analysis of WHO mortality database. Arthritis Rheum. 2017 Apr 20 [cited 2017 Jun 24]. Accepted manuscript online: DOI: 10.1002/art.40091

[69] Gabriel S. Rheumatoid arthritis in real life: How do you treat to target in 2016? American College of Rheumatology annual scientific meeting. 2016 Nov 14 [cited 2014 Mar 4]. Available from: http://acr.peachnewmedia.com/store/seminar/seminar.php?seminar=84767

[70] Olson A, Swigris JJ, Sprunger DB, Fischer A, Fernandez-Perez ER, Solomon J, Murphy J, Cohen M, Raghu G, Brown KK. Rheumatoid arthritis–interstitial lung disease–associated mortality. Am J Resp Crit Care. 2011 Feb [cited 2012 July 20];183(3):372-378. Available from: http://ajrccm.atsjournals.org/content/183/3/372.full DOI: 10.1164/rccm.201004-0622OC

[71] Laakso M, Isomäki H, Mutru O, Koota K. Death certificate and mortality in rheumatoid arthritis [abstract]. Scand J Rheumatol. 1986 [cited 2012 July 20];15(2):129-33. Available from: http://www.ncbi.nlm.nih.gov/pubmed/3749825

[72] Pincus T, Callahan LF, Sale WG, Brooks AL, Payne LE, Vaughn WK. Severe functional declines, work disability, and increased mortality in seventy-five rheumatoid arthritis patients studied over nine years. Arthritis Rheum. 1984 [cited 2016 Mar 5];27:864-872. Available from: http://www.ncbi.nlm.nih.gov/pubmed/6431998

[73] Abruzzo JL. Rheumatoid arthritis and mortality. Arthritis Rheum. 1982 Aug [cited 2016 Mar 5];25(8):1020-1023. Available from: http://onlinelibrary.wiley.com/doi/10.1002/art.1780250819/abstract

[74] Allebeck P, Ahlbom A, Allander E. Increased mortality among persons with rheumatoid arthritis, but where RA does not appear on death certificate: Eleven-year follow-up of an epidemiological study [abstract]. Scand J Rheumatol. 1981 [cited 2016 Mar 5];10(4):301-6. Available from: http://www.ncbi.nlm.nih.gov/pubmed/7323787

[75] Peltomaa R, Paimela L, Kautiainen H, Leirisalo-Repo M. Mortality in patients with rheumatoid arthritis treated actively from the time of diagnosis. Ann Rheum Dis. 2002 Apr [cited 2012 Jul 20]; 61:889-894. Available from: http://ard.bmj.com/content/61/10/889.full doi:10.1136/ard.61.10.889

[76] Pincus T. The paradox of effective therapies but poor long-term

outcomes in rheumatoid arthritis. Semin Arthritis Rheum. 1992 Jun [cited 2016 Mar 5]21(6):2-15 Suppl 3.

[77] Boers et al. Making an impact on mortality in rheumatoid arthritis. (See footnote Chapter 3.)

[78] Molina et al. Mortality in rheumatoid arthritis. (See footnote Chapter 3.)

[79] Gold LS, Ward MH, Dosemeci M, De Roos AJ. Systemic autoimmune disease mortality and occupational exposures. Arthritis Rheum. 2007 Oct [cited 2012 July 20];56(10):3189–3201. Available from: http://onlinelibrary.wiley.com/doi/10.1002/art.22880/full DOI:10.1002/art.22880

[80] Young A, Koduri G, Batley M, Kulinskaya E, Gough A, Norton S, Dixey J on behalf of the Early Rheumatoid Arthritis Study (ERAS) group. Mortality in rheumatoid arthritis. Increased in the early course of disease, in ischaemic heart disease and in pulmonary fibrosis. (Oxford) Rheumatology. 2007 Aug [cited 2012 July 20]; 46(2):350-357. Available from: http://rheumatology.oxfordjournals.org/content/46/2/350.full DOI: 10.1093/rheumatology/kel253

[81] Sacks JJ, Helmick CG, Langmaid G. Deaths from arthritis and other rheumatic conditions, United States, 1979-1998. J Rheumatol. 2004 Sep [cited 2013 Jun 22];31(9):1823-8. Available from: http://www.jrheum.org/content/31/9/1823.long

[82] Laakso et al. Death certificate and mortality. (See footnote Chapter 3.)

[83] Minaur NJ, Jacoby RK, Cosh JA, Taylor G, Rasker JJ. Outcome after 40 years with rheumatoid arthritis: A prospective study of function, disease activity, and mortality. J Rheumatol Suppl. 2004 Mar [cited 2016 Mar 5];69:3-8. Available from: http://jrheum.com/

subscribers/04/03supp/3.html

[84] Lindahl B. In what sense is rheumatoid arthritis the principal cause of death? A study of the National Statistics Office's way of reasoning based on 1224 death certificates [abstract]. J Chron Dis. 1985 [cited 2012 Sep 30];38(12):963-72. Available from: http://www.ncbi.nlm.nih.gov/pubmed/4066892

[85] Koivuniemi R, Paimela L, Leirisalo-Repo M. Causes of death in patients with rheumatoid arthritis from 1971 to 1991 with special reference to autopsy. Clin Rheumatol. 2009 Dec [cited 2012 Sep 30]; 28(12):1443-1447. Available from: http://www.springerlink.com/content/663137449n52777g/ DOI: 10.1007/s10067-009-1278-9

[86] Koivuniemi R. Causes of death in patients with rheumatoid arthritis over a 40-year period with special emphasis on autopsy [dissertation]. Helsinki (FI): Helsinki University; 2009 [cited 2013 May 4]. Available from: https://helda.helsinki.fi/bitstream/handle/10138/22895/causesof.pdf?sequence=1

[87] Listing J, Kekow J, Manger B, Burmester GR, Pattloch D, Zink A, Strangfeld A. Mortality in rheumatoid arthritis: The impact of disease activity, treatment with glucocorticoids, TNFα inhibitors and rituximab. Ann Rheum Dis. 2013 Dec 2 [cited 2016 Mar 5];0:1–7. DOI: 10.1136/annrheumdis-2013-204021

[88] Pincus et al. Severe functional declines. (See footnote Chapter 3.)

[89] Minaur et al. Outcome after 40 years with rheumatoid arthritis. (See footnote Chapter 3.)

[90] Molina et al. Mortality in rheumatoid arthritis. (See footnote Chapter 3.)

[91] Molina et al. Mortality in rheumatoid arthritis. (See footnote Chapter 3.)

[92] Molina et al. Mortality in rheumatoid arthritis. (See footnote Chapter 3.)

[93] Young K. How many people have rheumatoid arthritis? Rheumatoid Arthritis Warrior [website]. 2013 Mar 13 [cited 2013 May 4]. Available from: http://rawarrior.com/how-many-people-have-rheumatoid-arthritis/

[94] Gabriel SE, Michaud K. Epidemiological studies in incidence, prevalence, mortality, and comorbidity of the rheumatic diseases. Arthritis Res Ther. 2009 May 19 [cited 2013 Mar 12];11:229. Available from: http://arthritis-research.com/content/11/3/229 DOI:10.1186/ar2669

[95] Myasoedova E, Crowson CS, Kremers HM, Therneau TM, Gabriel SE. Is the incidence of rheumatoid arthritis rising? Results from Olmsted County, Minnesota, 1955-2007. Arthritis Rheum. 2010 [cited 2013 Mar 13];62(6):1576–1582. Available from: http://onlinelibrary.wiley.com/doi/10.1002/art.27425/full DOI: 10.1002/art.27425

[96] Centers for Disease Control and Prevention. [website]. Rheumatoid arthritis. 2012 Nov 19 [cited 2013 Apr 28]. Available from: http://www.cdc.gov/arthritis/basics/rheumatoid.htm

[97] Ruderman E, Tambar S. Rheumatoid arthritis. American College of Rheumatology [website]. 2012 Aug [cited 2013 Mar 13]. Available from: http://www.rheumatology.org/practice/clinical/patients/diseases_and_conditions/ra.asp

[98] Arthritis Foundation. Rheumatoid arthritis fact sheet. (See footnote Chapter 1.)

[99] 23 And Me [website]. About rheumatoid arthritis. 2009 Oct 4 [cited 2013 Mar 13]. Available from: https://www.23andme.com/health/Rheumatoid-Arthritis/

[100] Symmons D, Mathers C, Bruce Pfleger B. The global burden of rheumatoid arthritis in the year 2000. World Health Organization [website]. 2006 Aug 15 [cited 2013 Mar 13]. Available from: http://www.who.int/healthinfo/statistics/bod_rheumatoidarthritis.pdf

[101] Dave. Blazer's Edge Mailbag: Stats and their proper uses. Blazer's Edge [website]. 2013 Mar 6 [cited 2013 Mar 13]. Available from: http://www.blazersedge.com/2013/3/6/4069874/blazers-edge-mailbag-stats-sloan-sports-analystics-conference

CHAPTER FOUR
1st Evidence of Danger: Pre-clinical RA

Behind the mask of arthritis, pre-clinical disease is an early indication of health dangers

Pre-clinical disease activity

Rheumatoid disease is often referred to as an invisible illness since most symptoms are visibly subtle to casual observers.[1] However, the disease process is only invisible to the naked human eye. Disease activity is present in ways that medicine has lacked means to observe until recently with expert analysis of blood markers and skilled use of imaging equipment such as Doppler ultrasound.[2]

People eventually diagnosed with RA often describe years of symptoms that are currently attributable to the disease. Investigators have begun to uncover what is occurring invisibly during those years. "The presence of elevated serum levels of autoantibodies such as rheumatoid factors and antibodies to citrullinated proteins may precede the clinical onset of RA by over 10 years..."[3]

"The clinical onset of RA" refers to arthritis that is clinically diagnosable using specified criteria that emphasize synovial swelling of so-called small joints (usually MCPs). However, the disease is present and active within the body before it has generated suitable visible disease activity to satisfy the current diagnostic criteria for RA. Investigators who have explored the "preclinical phase of RA"[4] observed an accumulation of multiple autoantibodies that are evidence of "epitope expansion," a process which correlates closely with preclinical inflammation. "These antibodies and inflammatory cytokines are present years prior to the onset of symptoms in RA, suggesting that the autoimmune processes leading to arthritis are present long before overt disease manifestations."

Other investigators also refer to a "prearticular" period of RA in which musculoskeletal symptoms, again, do not satisfy diagnostic criteria, but disease activity has commenced within the patient's body: "The clinical manifestations in RA are preceded by a prodromal phase. This prearticular period is characterized by the presence of anti–citrullinated peptide/protein autoantibodies (anti–cyclic citrullinated peptide (anti-CCP)) and rheumatoid factor (RF), lipid dysregulation, and cardiovascular comorbidity."[5]

In 2013, van Steenbergen et al. reviewed studies from 2000 to 2012 on the "preclinical phase of RA."[6] According to van Steenbergen, EULAR has identified six non-linear phases of rheumatoid disease in order to better discuss and investigate "pre–RA." They acknowledge the protracted process of rheumatology recognizing "pre-RA" and "that disease processes related to RA occur before arthritis is clinically detectable was proposed more than two decades ago."

> "THERE IS A GROWING BODY OF EVIDENCE TO SUGGEST THAT AUTOIMMUNITY IN PATIENTS WITH RHEUMATOID ARTHRITIS (RA) IS INITIATED OUTSIDE THE JOINT."
>
> 2016, MIKULS ET AL.

(Footnote.)[7]

Lung evidence for pre-RA

Fischer et al. examined 74 patients with lung disease and no previous diagnosis of RA or similar connective tissue disease.[8] They noted a resemblance between the "lung phenotypic characteristics" of their patients and those with established RA. Additionally, approximately ten percent of their patients with lung disease and high levels of ACPA (three of thirty-three) developed joint symptoms sufficient to meet diagnostic criteria for RA within seven to eighteen months.

They suggest their results raise "suspicion that the lung disease in the subjects in our cohort may represent a forme fruste of RA —or perhaps a 'prearthritis' phenotype in the natural history of RA development."[9] A forme fruste presentation of RA would be an incomplete form of RA (like lung symptoms without joint symptoms). The term is usually used when "a well defined clinical or pathological entity,"[10] is only partially developed. It is hard to know what partially developed RA is, since neither its onset nor its fully developed form (full blown or "forme pleine"[11]) has been effectively defined. As previously discussed, investigators have only recently begun to establish the full scope of the disease, and current diagnostic criteria still do not take extra-articular disease into account.

A 2016 Karolinska University review asked the obvious question: "The lung in rheumatoid arthritis, cause or consequence?" It considers 66 research articles that examine the role of the lung in the development of rheumatoid disease.[12]

Chatzidionisyou et al. found all parts of the respiratory tract can be involved in RA. More importantly, they also established that respiratory tissue changes occur in early RA as often as with longstanding disease, "suggesting a potential role for these changes in the early stages of disease development."

They discuss several studies offering evidence about the significant and "early role of the adaptive immunity and immune activation in the lungs" of people with rheumatoid disease. The findings of their extensive review were compatible with a rheumatoid disease process that occurs in the lungs before symptoms are diagnosable in joints. They conclude that recognition of initiation of rheumatoid disease outside of the joints is an exciting development with important implications for further research.

Concurrently, Mikuls et al. reviewed several reports investigating mucosal sites such as lung and oral regions as "possible initiating sites for RA."[13] They "summarize recent reports incriminating these mucosal tissues as the initial site of autoantibody generation and inflammation in patients with RA." They maintain that "reports of pulmonary involvement preceding articular symptoms" in people with seropositive RA emphasize that the disease may be initiated in the lung. This notion is supported by the presence of antibodies highly specific to RA detected years before joint symptoms lead to a diagnosis of RA.

They conclude: "Overall, these studies support that RA-related autoimmunity can be generated in the lung in some subjects who do not have articular RA, perhaps as part of a natural response to local factors." The question is, if patients do not have "articular RA" (articular arthritis), what do they have? Since "articular" means "related to joints" and "arthritis" literally means inflamed joints," Mikuls et al. seem to state that the patients studied have arthritis that is not articular or "non-joint joint inflammation."

Stated more clearly, they have a disease that is not yet articular; they have rheumatoid disease.

Moreover, elevated anti-citrullinated peptide antibodies (ACPA), highly specific to RD, have been detected in the sputum (respiratory mucus) of first-degree relatives (FDRs) of people with rheumatoid disease who have not yet developed "classifiable RA."[14] Demoruelle et al. hypothesize that "local airway inflammation and NET (neutrophil extracellular traps) formation may drive anti-CCP production in the lung and may promote the early stages of RA development." They found ACPAs in the sputum of FDR's who were serum-negative for the antibodies, confirming that ACPAs can be present in lungs even earlier than in blood. This study is supportive of the theory that RD is initiated at a mucosal site (like the lungs) and confirms the need for further study of the process of development of RD, prior to the presence of overt arthritis.

SIGNIFICANCE OF PRE-CLINICAL RA

Acknowledgement of disease activity before or apart from swollen fingers (arthritis) is important for at least three reasons. Expanding the conception of rheumatoid disease beyond the notion of arthritis serves each of these urgent purposes.

> "GIVEN THE DEBILITATING NATURE AND CHRONICITY OF THESE CONDITIONS, PREVENTION OF AUTOIMMUNE RHEUMATIC DISEASE IS THE 'HOLY GRAIL.'"
>
> 2013, TUGNET ET AL.

(Footnote.)[15]

REASON ONE: Improved care for lower mortality

Most people in the medical field were trained with an understanding of RA that does not incorporate extra-articular disease. However, as rheumatologist Stephen Paget points out, "Rheumatic diseases (e.g., RA, SLE) affect the whole patient, not just the joints, and are associated with significant comorbidity and early mortality."[16] Studies of preclinical RA underscore the systemic nature of the disease and the need for a comprehensive approach to treatment and care of patients that includes addressing extra-articular problems.

Patient complaints of extra-articular symptoms often go unaddressed, one reason that the mortality rate of RD has not significantly improved. Mortality is essentially linked to extra-articular disease, and extra-articular symptoms are essentially linked to systemic disease activity.[17, 18, 19, 20] Patient care and mortality rates will improve as medical professionals are made more aware of the need to address extra-articular disease. Chapter 12 provides specific changes that can improve the quality of research and clinical care for patients.

Fatigue is a good example: As many as ninety percent of patients report experiencing disease-related fatigue[21] and experts rate it as a core disease measure.[22] This symptom could be dismissed as subjective and non-specific, as I have often seen, or medical explanations for fatigue could be explored, as is usually deemed appropriate in non-rheumatoid patients. Plausible causes of disease-related fatigue include anemia, decreased oxygen as a result of pulmonary issues, vitamin D deficiency, elevated white cell count, and cardiovascular involvement. A recent study of PRD without known cardiovascular disease showed that people with RD have heightened aortic wall inflammation and similar levels of carotid wall inflammation when compared to coronary artery disease patients without autoimmune disease.[23]

One way to help reduce mortality in PRD will be to make clinicians more aware that patient reports of systemic symptoms (such as fatigue) are potentially significant indicators.

REASON TWO: Improved research for better treatments

All clinical trials for prospective RD treatments and currently approved disease treatments are tested based upon measures of disease activity that are focused on conspicuous swelling of particular joints. PRD with obvious extra-articular features, viewed as comorbidities, are usually excluded from trials. Yet, these treatments are then prescribed for entire populations of PRD, regardless of extra-articular disease.

As mentioned above, a majority of patients have an inadequate response to those treatments. Recognition of extra-articular disease activity could broaden perspective in medical development to a more comprehensive approach, which could lead to treatment innovation. According to Deane and Mikuls, "The picture of RA etiology that is emerging leads us to inquire whether it and similar autoimmune conditions may eventually become preventable diseases, with prevention approaches focusing perhaps on mucosal inflammation and infection, rather than on joint disease."[24]

An ideal approach to RA treatment would be to arrest the onset of the disease in this preclinical phase; however, this is not yet possible. Advances in weighting the genetic and environmental determinants of autoimmunity in RA would increase the precision in predicting imminent onset of the disease, thereby allowing attempts at preventive interventions."[25]

Such a dramatic change in the understanding of the nature of rheumatoid disease and how it develops will likely bring a cure nearer.

REASON THREE: Improved diagnosis for increased remissions

As early as 1960, some investigators acknowledged that joint symptoms do not mark the initiation of rheumatoid disease: "Another difficulty ought to be touched upon: the onset of articular symptoms does not mark the onset of the disease process in a case of rheumatoid arthritis."[26] Fifty-two years later, Arend and Firestein declared: "Clinical RA is usually chronic by the time it is diagnosed and is preceded by an asymptomatic phase of unknown duration."[27] If they are right, it is imperative that pre-clinical disease is better understood in order to allow earlier diagnosis. Earlier diagnosis has proven the most effective way to increase the likelihood of remission with currently available treatments.

It is crucial to understand what is implied by the term "pre-clinical." Pre-clinical RA does not necessarily denote the time before any symptoms are present. Pre-clinical describes a person who may have musculoskeletal symptoms or even seek medical advice, but does not have *symptoms that fit the current diagnostic criteria for RA* in the subjective opinion of a particular clinician. Pre-clinical, in the case of RA, suggests "pre-articular," and specifically, before hand swelling is visibly evident to a rheumatologist (foot swelling can be substituted according to recent guideline revisions, but most doctors were trained with the hand paradigm). As discussed in Chapter 1, patients report that any joint or one of many systemic symptoms can be the first noticeable symptom of RD.[28]

I have received thousands of communications about this from patients, many of whom received medical care and even surgery for symptoms that are eventually attributed to RD—all before diagnosis. A characteristic example published by Mayo Clinic is the story of Sandy Blue who saw eight eye specialists over six months before finally traveling to Mayo Clinic where their "team approach" allowed her to be diagnosed with RA.[29] Sandy's first apparent symptom of the disease was scleritis, which inflamed her eyes so badly she could not see. She then responded to RD treatment.

Feedback from large numbers of patients causes me to suspect that eye symptoms, like other extra-articular symptoms, are not rare. The use of the word "rare" in the title of the preceding Mayo Clinic article is suggestive of the predicament of patients whose first RD symptom is not swollen hands. As long as the disease is designated as "arthritis," diagnosis will be delayed for many. The name "rheumatoid arthritis" perpetuates misguided notions that extra-articular symptoms are rare and typically occur later in the disease process. Recognition of pre-clinical disease could impel a more global approach to diagnosis.

Statistics quoted in the next two chapters will reveal that the impact of RD beyond the joints—including *10 Dangers of Rheumatoid Disease*—is not rare. And while I have waded through hundreds of medical journal articles in writing this book, footnoting many, a brief commentary from my blog at RA Warrior shows the significance of this research for individual people living with RD:

The following passage is adapted from an article on rawarrior.com, written in 2012.[30]

PRECLINICAL RHEUMATOID DISEASE: THERE ARE NO JOINTS IN THE LUNGS

My mom used to read to me John Godfrey Saxe's 19th century version of the famous Indian parable *The Blind Men and the Elephant.*[31] I'm certain it contributed to my zealous love of evidence. In the story, seven blind men encounter different aspects of the elephant, like the tusk, ear, or tail, and declare the elephant is very much like a spear, fan, or rope, respectively. The men disagree vehemently based on their partial experiences.

Over the last couple of years, interacting with thousands of people with rheumatoid disease, I came to the conclusion that only certain parts of this particular elephant were perceptible to those who define and treat the disease. Then, interacting with researchers, I saw that other parts of it are being identified behind the scenes. Today, I can bring you a glimpse of what we've witnessed.

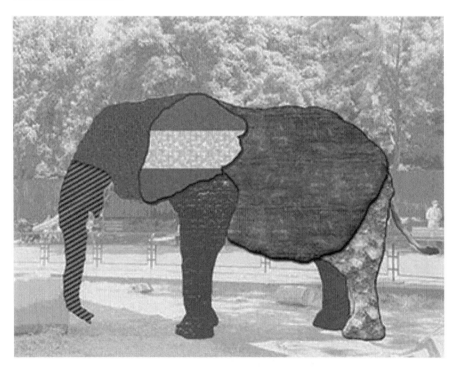

Bruce Jancin, staff writer for *Rheumatology News*, wrote about one of those parts in "Airways Abnormalities May Represent Preclinical Rheumatoid Arthritis."[32]

"Increasing *evidence suggests that RA is smoldering in the lungs during this preclinical stage, which can last a decade or more.* Indeed, bronchiole-associated lymphoid tissue may actually be the site where tolerance is broken and RA-related autoimmunity and systemic inflammation are generated, according to Dr. William F.C. Rigby, professor of medicine and professor of microbiology and immunology at Dartmouth Medical School, Hanover, NH...

"He credited the discovery of the existence of a *lengthy preclinical seropositive phase of RA* to landmark studies involving U.S. military personnel with centrally stored blood samples that were available for many years prior to their being diagnosed with RA (Ann. Rheum. Dis. 2008;67:801-7). The existence of this years-long preclinical lag time has since been confirmed in multiple other populations."

Preclinical RA in research and the real world

A week ago, when I was in Houston, I had lunch with a patient from Denver explaining that close to her home investigators are studying preclinical RA[33] by locating people with positive antibodies who do not yet have joint symptoms. Families like these want to know whether relatives (twins in this case!) will be affected. I described the strategy to observe what happens with RA before joints are affected. Four days later, we read the *Rheumatology News* article.

The Colorado researchers have been screening and conducting interviews with first-degree relatives of RA patients and obtaining blood samples[34] at community health fairs during the past few years learning to identify early RA and preclinical RA. According to Jancin, the earlier Armed Forces study demonstrated that the serologic profile method (anti-CCP and/or two or more rheumatoid factor isotopes) is 96% reliable for identifying RA before inflammatory arthritis is evident. We've examined possible triggers to rheumatoid disease, and you can see the advantage of being able to follow people who do not yet have diagnosable RA symptoms.

Airway disease exists prior to inflammatory arthritis symptoms

CT scans showed 77% of 45 preclinical RA patients experienced a form of airway disease. Only 31% of the antibody negative control group showed airway abnormality, but 12 people with early RA (diagnosed less than one year) were similar to the antibody positive pre-RA group.

Significantly, the found "none of the seropositive preclinical RA subjects with CT lung abnormalities had any evidence of synovitis of their joints on MRI, indicating that RA isn't necessarily smoldering pre-clinically in their joints for a long time prior to the time they show up in a rheumatologist's office with joint symptoms." In order to determine where RA disease begins and how to arrest it, we must look outside the joints as these researchers are. "These findings suggest that the lung may be an early site of autoimmune-related injury, and potentially a site of generation of RA-related autoimmunity. Further studies are needed to define the mechanistic role of lung inflammation in the development of RA."[35]

Commentary

We've known that joints are where rheumatoid disease ends up, but not likely where the disease begins. My unique vantage point, listening to the voices of so many people with this disease, has compelled me to advocate for research and treatment that considers the entire disease. We have yet to find the *sine qua non* of RD. But the future is rapidly arriving when we'll look at this elephant with our eyes wide open. At the very least each blind man's voice will be heard.

When I wrote that article in 2012, I knew from contacts with tens of thousands of patients and personal experiences with the disease that arthritis is only one symptom of RD. Since then, the Rheumatoid Patient Foundation has actually popularized that notion and even used it on a billboard: "arthritis is only one symptom." However, I have not been able to tell PRD what exactly to watch for. This book is the first such effort to document those concerns for patients. It grew from goals described in the blog excerpt above: to bring awareness of "extra-articular" aspects of RD and ultimately to save lives.

WHAT IS EXTRA-ARTICULAR DISEASE?

Extra-articular rheumatoid disease refers to symptoms beyond "arthritis."[36] Many such aspects of rheumatoid disease that are frequently experienced by patients have been confirmed by scientific study. However, this research has not yet penetrated most medical textbooks, schools, or websites. Therefore clinicians do not usually recognize these disease aspects because they expect only "arthritis" (joint inflammation). Most doctors who read this book will be better informed of the scope of this disease. As we connect the dots for the very first time, patients can seek more comprehensive care for their RD. And as these facts become more widely known, we should all anticipate progress, especially in reduced mortality, similar to what has been seen in recent decades with diabetes, SLE, and cancer.

Despite what is commonly taught in medical schools, and what patients are commonly told, extra-articular manifestations of the disease have been shown to be typical. That 1970's report, quoted earlier, found: "a high early incidence of extra-articular features in rheumatoid disease with 94 out of 102 patients showing manifestations in the 4.5 years from onset. This was so even though there was no bias towards severity in the sample, which included patients who had possible and probable disease as well as those with definite and classical disease. Only 8% showed no systemic manifestations and 41% had four or more."[37] They found extra-articular features in 92% of early RD cases despite lack of MRI, ultrasound, or HRCT (high-resolution computerized tomography) technology, and without considering CVD.

10 DANGERS OF RHEUMATOID DISEASE

The next chapters will describe ten areas in which health is threatened as a result of RD. Some dangers have only come to light in recent years, but others have been long recognized. It has been over 200 years that cardiovascular disease has been investigated in connection with RD. In most cases, a gradual recognition has occurred within a particular specialty such as pulmonology, without becoming part of common knowledge about the disease. Therefore, extra-articular aspects of the disease are not commonly measured or considered as part of rheumatological evaluations for either diagnosis or disease activity.

Over many years researchers from various medical specialties have studied these aspects of systemic RD separately, but these problems have never been measured together to calculate a complete picture of the risk that is experienced by a single PRD for RD-related serious illness or death. People with RD who have medical concerns relating to these or other extra-articular problems must seek care from each respective specialty. Unfortunately, even some doctors within a specialty may remain unaware of current research or of how to address these problems in RD.

We will explore the following list of serious and widespread aspects of the disease that every person living with RD must be aware of. However the reader ought bear in mind that the examples in this book are not exhaustive; other manifestations of systemic rheumatoid disease certainly exist. I have not conducted any explicit clinical study to produce this list. Yet, this book breaks new ground in simply compiling this list from published medical literature.

1. Oral Involvement

2. Laryngeal Involvement

3. Cardiovascular Involvement

4. Skin: rashes, vitiligo, Raynaud's

5. Constitutional symptoms: including fever, fatigue, and muscle wasting (cachexia), infections

6. Rheumatoid vasculitis and blood vessel disease

7. Lung Involvement

8. Kidney involvement

9. Eye involvement

10. Other organs: including spleen, liver, lymph system, gut

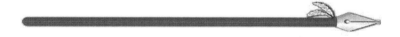

KEY POINTS

1. Some symptoms and antibodies can precede diagnosis over 10 years.

2. Many studies indicate RD begins in the lungs, before joint symptoms are diagnosable.

3. RD is often called an "invisible" illness because symptoms are not obvious to casual observers.

4. Doctors must be more aware that systemic symptoms like fatigue may indicate serious problems.

5. Extra-articular disease has been proven to affect most PRD, but is still not widely recognized.

6. Acknowledging rheumatoid disease that exists beyond and before joint inflammation (arthritis) could bring

    a) Improved care for lower mortality

    b) Improved research for better treatments

    c) Improved diagnosis for increased remissions

Action step: If you or a loved one has very early RA, find a doctor who will start observation and treatment as soon as possible to attempt to prevent onset of full-blown disease.

Quote to remember: One way to help reduce mortality in PRD will be to make clinicians more aware that patient reports of systemic symptoms (such as fatigue) are potentially significant indicators.

-----

[1] Copen L. Talking to someone with a chronic illness. CNN Health [website] 2012 Sep 11 [cited 2013 Apr 27]. Available from: http://www.cnn.com/2012/09/11/health/invisible-chronic-illness

[2] Brown AK, Emery P, et al. Presence of significant synovitis in rheumatoid arthritis patients with disease-modifying antirheumatic

drug–induced clinical remission. (See footnote Chapter 3.)

[3] Arend WP, Firestein GS. Pre-rheumatoid arthritis: Predisposition and transition to clinical synovitis. Nat Rev Rheumatol. 2012 Aug [cited 2012 Sep 30];8, 573–586. Available from: http://www.nature.com/nrrheum/journal/v8/n10/full/nrrheum.2012.134.html

[4] Sokolove J, Bromberg R, Deane KD, Lahey LJ, Derber LA, Chandra PE, Edison JD, Gilliland WR, Tibshirani RJ, Norris JM, et al. Autoantibody epitope spreading in the pre-clinical phase predicts progression to rheumatoid arthritis. PLoS One. 2012 May [cited 2012 Sep 30];7(5):e35296. Available from: http://www.plosone.org/article/info%3Adoi%2F10.1371%2Fjournal.pone.0035296 doi: 10.1371/journal.pone.0035296

[5] Colmegna et al. Current understanding of rheumatoid arthritis therapy. (See footnote in Introduction.)

[6] van Steenbergen HW, et al. Review: The preclinical phase of rheumatoid arthritis: What is acknowledged and what needs to be assessed? (See footnote Chapter 3.)

[7] Mikuls TR, Payne JB, Deane KD, Thiele GM. Autoimmunity of the lung and oral mucosa in a multisystem inflammatory disease: The spark that lights the fire in rheumatoid arthritis? J Allergy Clin Immunol. 2016 Jan [cited 2017 Jun 25];137(1):28-34. Available from: http://www.jacionline.org/article/S0091-6749(15)01581-X/fulltext

[8] Fischer et al. Lung disease with anti-CCP antibodies but not rheumatoid arthritis or connective tissue disease. (See footnote Chapter 1.)

[9] Fischer et al. Lung disease with anti-CCP antibodies but not rheumatoid arthritis or connective tissue disease. (See footnote

Chapter 1.)

[10] Wikipedia contributors. Forme fruste. Wikipedia, The Free Encyclopedia [Internet]; 2017 Feb 22[cited 2017 Jul 1]. Available from: https://en.wikipedia.org/w/index.php?title=Forme_fruste&oldid=766760023

[11] Wikipedia. Forme fruste. (See footnote Chapter 4.)

[12] Chatzidionisyou A, Catrina AI. The lung in rheumatoid arthritis, cause or consequence? Curr Opin Rheumatol. 2016 Jan [cited 2017 Mar 19];28(1):76–82. DOI:10.1097/BOR.0000000000000238

[13] Mikuls et al. Autoimmunity of the lung and oral mucosa in a multisystem inflammatory disease. (See footnote Chapter 4.)

[14] Demoruelle MK, Harrall KK, Ho L, Purmalek MM, Seto NL, Rothfuss HM, Weisman MH, Solomon JJ, Fischer A, Okamoto Y, et al. Anti–citrullinated protein antibodies are associated with neutrophil extracellular traps in the sputum in relatives of rheumatoid arthritis patients. Arthritis Rheum. 2017 Jun [cited 2017 June 25];69(6):1165–1175.DOI:10.1002/art.40066

[15] Tugnet et al. Human endogenous retroviruses (HERVs) and autoimmune rheumatic disease. (See footnote in Chapter 1.)

[16] Paget, S. Making a difference for rheumatoid arthritis patients: Early diagnosis and rapid referral. Rheumatoid arthritis primary care initiative for improved diagnosis and outcomes. Women in Government [website]. 2008 Sep [cited 2013 Apr 14]. Available from: http://www.womeningovernment.org/files/Microsoft%20PowerPoint%20-%20paget_ra_sept_2008.pdf

[17] Turesson C, O'Fallon WM, Crowson CS, Gabriel SE, Matteson EL. Extra-articular disease manifestations in rheumatoid arthritis: Incidence trends and risk factors over 46 years. Ann Rheum Dis. 2003 [cited 2013 Apr 27];62:722-727 Available from: http://

ard.bmj.com/content/62/8/722.full DOI:10.1136/ard.62.8.722

[18] Turan Y, KocaaĆa Z, Koçyiğit H, Gürgan A, Barış Bayram K, İpek S. Correlation of fatigue with clinical parameters and quality of life in rheumatoid arthritis. Turk J Rheumatol. 2010 [cited 2013 Apr 27]; 25: 63-7. Available from: http://romatizma.dergisi.org/pdf/ pdf_ART_346.pdf

[19] Ibn Yacoub Y, Amine B, Laatiris A, Wafki F, Znat F, Hajjaj-Hassouni N. Fatigue and severity of rheumatoid arthritis in Moroccan patients [abstract]. Rheumatol Int. 2012 Jul [cited 2013 Apr 27];32(7):1901-7. Available from: http://www.ncbi.nlm.nih.gov/ pubmed/21448644 DOI: 10.1007/s00296-011-1876-0

[20] Zoto A, Selimi B. Ocular involvement in patients with rheumatoid arthritis. Ophthalmology Research: An International Journal. 2015 Jun 19 [cited 2017 Mar 22];4(4): 99-103. Available from: http:// www.journalrepository.org/media/journals/OR_23/2015/Jun/ Zoto442015OR18637.pdf

[21] Rheumatoid Patient Foundation. Unmasking rheumatoid disease. (See Footnote Chapter 2.)

[22] Kirwan JR, Minnock P, Adebajo A, Bresnihan B, Choy E, de Wit M, Hazes M, Richards P, Saag K, Suarez-Almazor M, et al. Patient perspective: Fatigue as a recommended patient centered outcome measure in rheumatoid arthritis. J Rheumatol. 2007 May [cited 2013 Apr 27];34(5):1174-7. Available from: http://www.ncbi.nlm.nih.gov/ pubmed/17477482

[23] Greenberg JD, Fayad Z, Furer V, Farkouh M, Colin MJ, Rosenthal PB, Samuels J, Samuels SK, Reddy SM, Izmirly PM, et al. Heightened aortic wall inflammation in patients with rheumatoid arthritis versus patients with established coronary artery disease without autoimmune disease [abstract]. Arthritis Rheum. 2012 Oct [cited 2013 Apr 27];64(10 Supplement)#1250. Available from: http://

www.blackwellpublishing.com/acrmeeting/abstract.asp?
MeetingID=789&id=101970&meeting=ART201264

[24] Deane K. Preventing rheumatoid arthritis? (See footnote in
Chapter 1.)

[25] Colmegna et al. Current understanding of rheumatoid arthritis
therapy. (See footnote in Introduction.)

[26] Jonsson E. On the prognosis of rheumatoid arthritis. Acta
Orthopaedica Scandinavica. 1961 [cited 2013 Apr 13];30(1-4):
115-123. Available from: http://dx.doi.org/
10.3109/17453676109149531 DOI:10.3109/17453676109149531

[27] Arend WP. Pre-rheumatoid arthritis. (See footnote Chapter 4.)

[28] Young K. What is the first symptom of rheumatoid arthritis?
Rheumatoid Arthritis Warrior [website]. 2009 [cited 2013 Apr 14].
Available from: http://rawarrior.com/what-is-the-first-symptom-of-
rheumatoid-arthritis

[29] Rivas R. Rare arthritis no match for woman determined to save her
eyesight. Sharing Mayo Clinic: Stories from patients, family, friends
and Mayo Clinic staff [website]. 2012 Aug 23 [cited 2013 Apr 14].
Available from: http://sharing.mayoclinic.org/2012/08/23/rare-
arthritis-no-match-for-woman-determined-to-save-her-eyesight/

[30] Young K. Preclinical rheumatoid disease. (See footnote in Chapter
1.)

[31] Saxe JG. The blind men and the elephant [poem]. In: Linton WJ.
Poetry of America. 1878 Jan [cited 2012 Sep 30]. p 150-152.

[32] Jancin B. Airways abnormalities may represent preclinical
rheumatoid arthritis. Rheumatology News [website]. 2012 [cited
2012 Sep 30]. Available from: http://www.rheumatologynews.com/
single-view/airways-abnormalities-may-represent-preclinical-

rheumatoid-arthritis/06cf3d5ce6.html

[33] Demoruelle MK, Weisman MH, Simonian PL, Lynch DA, Sachs PB, Pedraza IF, Harrington AR, Kolfenbach JR, Striebich CC, Pham QN, et al. Brief report: Airways abnormalities and rheumatoid arthritis-related autoantibodies in subjects without arthritis: Early injury or initiating site of autoimmunity? Arthritis Rheum. 2012 Jun [cited 2012 Sep 30];64(6):1756–1761. Available from: http:// onlinelibrary.wiley.com/doi/10.1002/art.34344/full DOI: 10.1002/ art.34344

[34] Deane KD, Striebich CC, Goldstein BL, Derber LA, Parish MC, Feser ML, Hamburger EM, Brake S, Belz C, Goddard J, et al. Identification of undiagnosed inflammatory arthritis in a community health-fair screen. Arthritis Rheum. 2009 Dec 15 [cited 2012 Sep 30];61(12):1642–1649. Available from: http:// www.ncbi.nlm.nih.gov/pmc/articles/PMC2913880/ DOI: 10.1002/ art.24834

[35] Demoruelle et al. Brief report: Airways abnormalities. (See footnote Chapter 4.)

[36] Fleming A, Dodman S, et al. Extra-articular features in early rheumatoid disease. (See footnote in Chapter 1.)

[37] Fleming A, Dodman S, et al. Extra-articular features in early rheumatoid disease. (See footnote in Chapter 1.)

CHAPTER FIVE
DANGERS BEYOND JOINTS: MORE EVIDENCE OF RD

As RD attacks beyond the joints, its systemic nature is clear

Extra-articular disease is not a "complication"

The term "complication" is used in medicine to denote a problem that arises as a result of a separate cause than a diagnosis in question. According to this understanding, a runny nose could not be a complication of a cold because a runny nose is a symptom of a cold. An actual complication of a cold could be a sore nose resulting from use of rough facial tissues. In another example, complications of kidney surgery could arise through many causes such as hospital error, patient's infection, or equipment failure. But symptoms of the original kidney disease would not be called complications of the surgery.

Similarly, it is incorrect to regard extra-articular manifestations of RD as "complications" of the disease. Doing so says every dangerous problem caused by the disease has some separate cause. And more importantly, it makes the disease into a condition of joint inflammation only, or a form of arthritis, which is untrue. *Investigation of the evidence reveals a dangerous and complicated disease that is not limited to joint inflammation (arthritis).*

In their 2010 paper, Cojocaru et al. bluntly define extra-articular rheumatoid disease and the need for greater recognition of it: "Extra-articular manifestations are all the conditions and symptoms which are not directly related to the locomotor system."[1] They summarize several extra-articular manifestations of RD including epithelial (skin), ocular, oral, gastrointestinal, pulmonary, cardiac, renal, neurological, and hematological.

Their broad approach gives recognition to the association between the systemic aspects of RD and the morbidity and mortality of PRD: "The extra-articular manifestations of RA can occur at any age after onset. It is characterised by destructive polyarthritis and extra-articular organ involvement, including the skin, eye, heart, lung, renal, nervous and gastrointestinal systems. The frequency of extra-articular manifestations in RA differs from one country to another. Extra-articular organ involvement in RA is more frequently seen in patients with severe, active disease and is associated with increased mortality."[2]

We will now look individually at these manifestations.

ONE: Oral involvement

Periodontitis has been known to be statistically associated with RA. In recent years, several investigators have explored the relationship between the common oral bacteria Porphyromonas gingivalis (Pg) and the initiation of citrullination, a process involved in the development of RA. Citrullination is a process that converts part of a protein from arginine to citrulline. This process only changes one atom at the end of a protein, but the immune system of PRD recognizes that citrulline is not one of the naturally occurring amino acids, and it generates anti–citrullinated peptide antibodies (ACPAs). ACPAs are highly specific to RD (tested as anti-CCP).

This process is referred to as the "loss of tolerance," as the body attacks these citrullinated proteins that are a person's own cells. According to current theory, the immune system attacks these cells, no longer recognizing them as "self." The person experiences a loss of "self-tolerance." This is the beginning of auto-immunity. In some people the loss of self-tolerance occurs first in the mouth.

Totaro et al. built on and confirmed the work of others on the possibility of a free DNA transport to the joint compartment from the mouth, exploring the "possibility that oral bacteria or their genetic material could reach the joints." Indeed their data supported the "possibility that the genetic material was carried out from teeth to joints." Remarkably, no relationship was found between the presence of Pg DNA and common RD antibody (ACPA or RF) levels. And, confirming previous findings of other investigators, Pg DNA was more likely to be present in early rheumatoid disease rather than in later stage disease.[3]

Many have warned that this research suggests that PRD ought to take particular care of oral health to avoid worse disease. While there is not evidence to support this, a more important suggestion would be for close relatives of people with RD, who could be at higher risk, to be cautioned that oral inflammation may be a warning sign of possible developing RD. Further research in this area could contribute to the conception of an earlier method of testing for RD, that does not involve the joints.

People with RD often experience excessive mouth dryness. This can be caused by Sjögren's syndrome (discussed below) which frequently occurs in PRD. Sjögren's syndrome causes mouth dryness by impairing the function of exocrine glands.

> "THE PHONATORY AND AIRWAY SYMPTOMS ARE VERY OFTEN OVERLOOKED BY THE PHYSICIAN WHO IS MORE FOCUSED ON THE SEVERE SMALL JOINT POLYARTHROPATHY."
>
> 2007, HAMDEN ET AL.

(Footnote.)[4]

TWO: Laryngeal involvement

Inside the larynx are tiny cartilage bones; the cricoid and arytenoid together form the cricoarytenoid (CA) joint. RD can affect CA joints in various ways, causing erosion, inflammation, or nodules, resulting in vocal cord fixation or vocal cord immobility. This has become more widely recognized by patients since I have written about case studies and clinical research on CA on rawarrior.com for several years.

However, laryngeal involvement in RD can be much broader than CA joint inflammation. One investigator summarized the research in laryngeal involvement this way: "Laryngeal manifestations of rheumatoid arthritis may be in the form of laryngeal myositis, neuropathy of the recurrent laryngeal nerve, postcricoid granulomas, cricoarytenoid joint arthritis and rheumatic submucosal nodules."[5] Specific laryngoscopic findings have also included: "mucosal edema, myositis of the intrinsic laryngeal muscles, hyperemia, inflammation and swelling of the arytenoids, interarytenoid mucosa, aryepiglottic folds and epiglottis, and impaired mobility or fixation of the cricoarytenoid joint" and "inflammatory masses or rheumatoid nodules in the larynx and pharynx."[6]

Vocal cord immobility can cause symptoms which are usually annoying, and rarely, life threatening. Symptoms experienced by patients include hoarseness, change in range of voice, loss of voice, pain during speaking or swallowing, feeling of fullness or mass in the throat, choking sensation, shortness of breath, or difficulty breathing. Laryngeal involvement in the forms of both "laryngeal symptoms and laryngeal alterations are frequent in RA patients" when studied by patient questionnaires and videolaryngoscopy.[7] Visible CA inflammation has been shown to correlate with "active disease elsewhere in the body."[8]

In 1963, *Arthritis & Rheumatism*, a journal of the American College of Rheumatology, published a report from the Hospital for Special Surgery in New York with the following finding: "Arthritis of the cricoarytenoid joints occurs much more frequently in patients with rheumatoid disease than has been generally suspected. Persistent hoarseness is the most common symptom and evidence of inflammation and/or dysfunction of the cricoarytenoid joints can often be seen by indirect laryngoscopy. The correlated autopsy and clinical findings indicate that rheumatoid cricoarytenoid arthritis may exist in a clinically undetectable form."[9] Again, "clinically undetectable" does not necessarily imply patients are symptom-free; it refers to the inability of clinicians to consistently detect symptoms that meet certain criteria. And although the notion persists that CA involvement is rare in RD, multiple sources have repeatedly confirmed CA involvement in rheumatoid disease is frequent, occurring in 70 to 90 percent of patients.[10, 11, 12, 13, 14, 15]

Larynx involvement is a typical example of extra-articular disease in that the condition is common in patients, yet believed by most clinicians to be uncommon, and therefore seldom diagnosed or treated. One reason may be that findings of numerous studies show that it is not easily identified visibly, even with laryngoscope. However, more complex imaging, especially high-resolution computerized tomography (HRCT), corroborates what has been demonstrated with autopsy studies: that cricoarytenoid involvement in rheumatoid disease is not uncommon. Different methods of examination have differing levels of sensitivity to identify it: Bayar detected only 13.3% percent of patients with CA involvement using endoscopy, but 80% using HRCT in a group of patients where 66.6% had CA symptoms.[16]

According to Benggston, "Lack of knowledge about this disease in combination with the fact that there are many other causes leading to dyspnoea in the RA patient, is a probable reason for the condition's easily being overlooked. It is more likely to be diagnosed as 'asthma' or unspecific laryngitis. Arthritis of the cricoarytenoid joints is considered to be a rare cause of dyspnoea. It is somewhat surprising, therefore, that the prevalence ranges from 13-75% in different RA materials and between 45-88% in postmortem studies."[17] Hamden also notes that "clinical prevalence falls below the postmortem histopathological diagnosis of laryngeal involvement which is estimated to be up to 90% of the cases."[18]

Other areas of the throat may also be affected. In a study of PRD with advanced disease, eighty-two percent showed narrowing of the cricothyroid joint, with significant loss of voice range. Most patients experienced vocal fatigue and 36% experienced hoarseness.[19] Nodules and inflammation can develop elsewhere. "Furthermore, RA affects the ear, nose, and throat, causing various otorhinolaryngological symptoms... Although the ear and nose involvement in RA is relatively benign and uncommon, laryngeal RA manifestations are much more serious."[20] Systemic or extra-articular symptoms such as cricoarytenoid effects are not restricted to advanced disease and have occurred as the initial or single clinical manifestation of rheumatoid disease.[21, 22, 23, 24]

Lack of awareness of laryngeal involvement can have serious

consequences. In addition to the natural consequences of the disease, multiple investigators have historically noted that the condition may complicate anesthesia procedures[25] or may cause patients to experience loss of voice following anesthesia.[26] "The anesthesiologist should handle with extreme care the inflamed laryngeal structures and be least aggressive in securing the airway."[27] However, in large part due to designation of RD as a "type of arthritis," synovitis has been the principal, if not singular, concern of most doctors treating RD patients: "The phonatory and airway symptoms are very often overlooked by the physician who is more focused on the severe small joint polyarthropathy."[28] In a recent in-depth study of the topic, Iacovou et al. point out the urgency of doctors becoming more aware: "Not only should Rheumatologists be aware of laryngeal involvement in connective tissue disorders, but also ENT surgeons should be actively involved in the management of these patients, as such involvement may become life threatening."[29]

THREE: Cardiovascular involvement

In 1949, Bywaters discussed what was then a "classic article on Rheumatism of the Heart (1812) (which) gives the full story of a number of very pertinent cases illustrating this first association of heart and joint disease."[30] Bywaters was not alone in his interest in the heart disease of rheumatic patients; his article used fifty-seven references to other works. Articles written as early as 1812 and 1836 demonstrate an early consciousness of a connection between joint disease and heart disease. Investigators speculated whether rheumatoid disease was related to rheumatic fever when autopsies of PRD studied by several researchers revealed distinct cardiac changes in a third of cases.[31]

Autopsies were later used to demonstrate the nature of cardiac damage in PRD and refute any connection to rheumatic fever. A 1959 report identified "three different ways in which the heart may be affected by rheumatoid disease": *Rheumatoid Pericarditis, Rheumatoid Granuloma in the Heart*, and *Rheumatoid Arteritis*. It summarized: "A description is given of three patients with rheumatoid arthritis who died as a result of rheumatoid disease of the cardiovascular system. These three patients illustrate the occurrence of rheumatoid pericarditis, rheumatoid nodules in the heart and rheumatoid arteritis. These lesions are known to occur in rheumatoid arthritis and are not rheumatic (fever) in origin."[32]

By 1963, appreciation of RD as a systemic disease with potential for cardiac harm had taken hold, as evidenced by even the title of several articles, such as "Rheumatoid Heart Disease. A Case Study with Illustrations,"[33] "Cardiac Disease in Rheumatoid Arthritis"[34] and "The Heart in Rheumatoid Arthritis (Rheumatoid Disease): A Clinical and Pathological Study of Sixty-two Cases" which describes heart involvement as frequent and related to other disease manifestations. Lebowitz nevertheless bemoans the lack of credence yet given to cardiac symptoms.[35]

In 1969, Kirk and Cosh declared skepticism for the concept of rheumatoid heart disease: "Heart disease in a patient with rheumatoid arthritis is usually due to coincidental and unrelated pathology. However, true rheumatoid heart disease exists in two main forms, although its identification may be uncertain without knowledge of the morbid anatomy": granuloma and pericarditis. They claimed that incidence was more rare than what others supposed and that its manifestations are slight.[36]

Ultrasound was eventually available to confirm heart pathologies at rates similar to autopsies, allowing the conclusion that "(A)ll anatomical structures of the heart may be involved."[37] Frequency was still uncertain, but mortality was believed to be increased.

A 2004 report on premature mortality in RA found 42% of deaths in RA were due to cardiovascular causes, about the same as about three decades earlier.[38] It was the most common cause of death in RA. For comparison, about 25% of deaths in the general U.S. population are due to cardiovascular disease.[39] Manzi and Wasko observed a higher frequency of cardiovascular disease (CVD) in young females: "The most striking findings of increased mortality in RA due to coronary heart disease have been in young women aged 15–49, where SMRs (standard mortality ratios) are as high as 3.64."[40] (This indicates 3.64 times as many deaths per year as should be expected.)

In recent years, evidence has continued to mount for the existence of "rheumatoid heart disease" because "RD may confer risk independently" of traditional risk factors.[41] Through data from the Rochester Epidemiology Project, Mayo Clinic led the way in researching mortality of rheumatoid disease, which led them inevitably to rheumatoid heart disease.[42] They have demonstrated that risk assessment tools typically used to measure CVD risk often underestimate risk in PRD: "This indicates that RA disease severity and inflammation play a role in CVD risk that is not accounted for in the Framingham risk score. In addition, the Reynolds risk score underestimated CVD risk in women with RA, despite its inclusion of C-reactive protein."[43]

Another study published in the *Journal of the American College of Cardiology*, "Left Ventricular Systolic Dysfunction in Rheumatoid Disease: An Unrecognized Burden," investigated "whether left ventricular systolic dysfunction (LVSD) is more common among clinic patients with rheumatoid disease (RD) compared with the general population."[44] They found LVSD to be "three times more common in RD patients than in the general population." Forty-eight percent of PRD had electrocardiographic (ECG) abnormalities, an independent predictor of LVSD. Clinical evidence of ischemic heart disease (IHD) in almost half of cases and other findings led to the conclusion that further investigation would be valuable. Lack of prior research is a recognized problem: "However, studies detailing the coronary anatomy and nature of lesions in rheumatoid patients with IHD are surprisingly scarce, yet would be most valuable."

Recent years have brought numerous other investigations into left ventricular dysfunction in RD. Levendoglu et al. used Doppler recordings to measure performance of specific heart abnormalities in PRD. They found both ventricles were impaired in active RD. However, "There was a direct relationship between some of the parameters of left ventricular diastolic function and disease duration as well. These findings suggest a subclinical myocardial involvement in RA patients."[45] The intimation of a "subclinical" problem is crucial. This demonstrates that changes can be detected before symptoms are "clinically" diagnosable, which could have possible future implications for treatment. Their results also underscore the connection between disease duration and cardiac dysfunction.

The same year, Bharti et al. published an "Assessment of left ventricular systolic and diastolic function in juvenile rheumatoid arthritis."[46] They also found that patients who were "asymptomatic" for cardiac dysfunction nonetheless suffered significant systolic and diastolic functional abnormalities. Changes in the dimensions of the left ventricle were found to be the same as in adult RD. Diastolic dysfunction was common.

They concluded: "Despite an asymptomatic cardiac status, significant systolic and diastolic functional abnormalities exist in patients with JRA. The duration of the disease, mode of presentation, patient's age and gender have a significant impact on the left ventricular systolic and diastolic functions in patients with JRA."[47] They advocated closer monitoring of patients for more overt cardiac symptoms.

In 2007, Kelly and Hamilton found that ischemic heart disease accounted for a quarter of all deaths in RA.[48] It was the most common cause of "death at a young age." They found a relationship between disease activity and probability of death from IHD. That same year, Mayo Clinic published recommendations for a comprehensive cardiovascular risk assessment for all newly diagnosed PRD.[49]

In a 2009 letter to the editor, Vizzardi et al. discuss Rudominer's report on increased left ventricular (LV) mass in association with RA and their own study of "93 randomly enrolled RA patients," citing five related publications as well. They describe several distinctive CV effects of rheumatoid disease: "The stiffening of the aorta and other central arteries represents a potential risk factor for increased cardiovascular morbidity and mortality. Furthermore, an association between impaired aortic elasticity and LV hypertrophy has been demonstrated in previous studies. Our findings confirm those of Rudominer and colleagues and demonstrate an association between some aspects of impaired aortic elasticity and increased LV mass in RA patients. These findings suggest that patients with RA could have preclinical atherosclerosis, even without having hypertension or other cardiovascular risk factors. A decrease in aortic elasticity could influence the natural history of RA and contribute to the development of cardiovascular disease and left ventricular dysfunction."[50]

In 2010, investigators showed that in newly diagnosed PRD with no signs of atherosclerosis, endothelial dependent flow-mediated dilation (ED-FMD) and intima media thickness (IMT) "related to biomarkers known to be associated with endothelial dysfunction and atherosclerosis." And: "After 18 months, IMT had increased significantly in RA patients but not in controls." They concluded endothelial activation may be implicated very early in the disease process, preceding signs of endothelial dysfunction. "Considering the current state of knowledge, the necessity of optimising prevention and treatment of CVD in patients with RA must be emphasised."[51]

One of the most recent discoveries relates to changes in the shape or structure of the left ventricle, called remodeling, usually caused by heart injury or heart disease. Mayo Clinic researchers found "RA was strongly associated with abnormal LV remodeling, particularly, with concentric LV remodeling, among patients without HF (heart failure). This association was significant beyond adjustment for cardiovascular risk factors and comorbidities. RA disease related factors may promote changes in LV geometry. The biological mechanisms underlying LV remodeling warrant further investigation."[52]

Angina, a painful tight sensation caused by reduced blood flow to the heart, is one of the few CVD problems which has not been widely demonstrated to be more common in PRD. However, Swedish investigators recently reported an increased RD risk of *acute coronary syndrome*.[53] This is an umbrella term that includes both heart attacks (MI) and angina. Experts have suggested that angina may be underestimated in RD because the pain PRD report with angina would seem similar to (shoulder) arthritis pain. This could lead to an assumption that the symptom is joint-related so that it is not investigated further.[54]

A separate dilemma is how to treat increased CVD risk in people with rheumatoid disease.

An "Unresolved Questions in Rheumatology" debate in 2013 focused on how to respond to this increased CVD risk.[55] Peters and Nurmohamed equated CVD risk in RA to that of type-1 diabetes, which has been more effectively addressed in recent decades with risk management strategies. However, with "RA, the magnitude of CVD has not appreciably changed over the last decades. Despite this well-established higher cardiovascular risk, a significant proportion of RA patients still receive no or suboptimal cardiovascular risk management. Based on this evidence, we can no longer bury our heads in the sand and pretend that cardiovascular risk management should not be part of our agenda." Proposals for addressing this problem include the creation of "CVD risk prediction charts" for RA. They explain, "This will take many years, however, and in the meantime, many patients will receive suboptimal cardiovascular risk management because existing CVD risk prediction charts underestimate the true cardiovascular risk in RA." Although studies have suggested that common tools such as the Framingham assessment (discussed above) underestimate CVD risk in RA by at least 50%, they "recommended that patients receive a yearly cardiovascular risk assessment" in the meantime.

Debating Peters and Nurmohamed, Dixon emphasized the need for guidelines in managing CVD risk in PRD, drawing attention to "15 new articles (that) have been published on this topic every month over the last 5 years." Dixon also stressed that it is not known how much increased CVD in PRD is attributable to disease factors such as inflammation versus traditional risk factors recognized in the general population such as lipid levels. Peters and Nurmohamed forcefully argue for the use of available medications such as statins or antihypertensive agents in PRD with higher CV risk, because despite the lack of specialized randomized clinical trials of these drugs in PRD, there is "no rationale for why chronic inflammation or other RA-related factors would render" those drugs ineffective.

All contributors agreed that more must be done to address CVD in RD, both in research investigation and in the clinical setting. Peters and Nurmohamed: "A recent study suggests that there is poor cardiovascular risk management by primary care physicians as well as rheumatologists. This clearly demonstrates the need for better education to improve awareness of cardiovascular risk in RA." While the research they debate is crucial, the education of physicians should be the simpler and shorter task that could better the outcomes of people living with rheumatoid disease. There was no debate over the necessity for that.

There are some positive indications of change toward greater awareness of CVD in RD, including the establishment of cardiac-rheumatology centers to better diagnose and treat PRD, such as the Preventive Cardio-Rheuma clinic at Diakonhjemmet Hospital in Oslo, Norway and Mayo Clinic's Cardio-Rheumatology Clinic.[56] The "emerging field of cardiorheumatology" has only begun to document the many CV manifestations in RD and explore appropriate recommendations for treating PRD.[57]

Also, while funding for RD research remains lower than for comparable diseases (see Chapter 8), the descriptions of a few NIH grants seem promising for progress in CVD of RD. Titles include: "Mechanisms Linking Joint Inflammation and Atherosclerosis in Rheumatoid Arthritis," "Heart Disease in Rheumatoid Arthritis," "Development of a Novel RA/

Atherosclerosis Mouse Model."[58]

Investigation of the incidence and risks of cardiovascular involvement is fundamental to improving outcomes of PRD.

Risks of specific CVD manifestations have been shown to exist, some already at the point of RD diagnosis. Recent research at Mayo Clinic confirms that CVD risk in RD "is independent of standard cardiovascular (CV) risk factors and correlates with RA disease activity."[59] It is imperative to learn how the disease process leads to such risks. This is the crucial work of investigators who ask: What makes PRD die prematurely, and how can it be stopped?

The following is a partial list of CVD manifestations of RD, encountered while researching this chapter: myocardial infarction (MI), death after first MI, silent MI, stroke, atrial fibrillation, left ventricular systolic dysfunction, left ventricular remodeling, cardiac lesions or nodules, aortitis, pericarditis, epicarditis, endocarditis, myocarditis, arteritis, left ventricle stiffening, ischemic heart disease (IHD), valvopathy, coronary artery risk increase, and increased atherosclerosis.

An entry from my blog at RA Warrior in 2011 succinctly lists several important facts related to rheumatoid heart disease:

The following passage is adapted from an article on rawarrior.com[60]

20 SPECIFIC FINDINGS ON RHEUMATOID HEART DISEASE

Reading dozens of studies has convinced me that rheumatoid heart disease is part of rheumatoid

disease. It is not simply...

- RA increasing a person's chances of heart disease.

- RA making heart disease worse.

- RA patients being more likely to die if they get heart disease.

Rather, it means...

1. Increased RA mortality can largely be attributed to increased cardiovascular death.

2. RA patients are twice as likely to experience unrecognized heart attacks and sudden cardiac deaths.

3. The increased risk of heart attack is already there at the time a RA diagnosis is first made.

4. Several traditional cardiovascular risk factors were found to behave differently in RA patients.

5. Cardiovascular risk scores for the general population may underestimate the risk for RA patients.

6. Optimal control of cardiovascular risk factors is important, but not sufficient in RA patients. RA-specific cardiovascular risk prediction tools are needed.

7. Dr. Maradit Kremers: "Something else is going on. It could be that rheumatoid arthritis and heart disease have a common origin."

8. Data support the hypothesis that a blood-based immunologic signature (IL-17) may be useful to identify patients at risk for adverse disease outcomes such as heart failure.

9. People with RA who experience sudden cardiac death are less likely to have had a history of chest pain than those without RA.

10. Increased cardiac events in RA patients could not be

explained by an increase in traditional heart disease risk factors such as elevated cholesterol, blood pressure and body mass index, diabetes, and alcohol abuse.

11. Heart disease can remain silent in those with RA. Regular cardiac checkups are important, as is lowering traditional cardiac risk factors such as taking care of blood pressure and cholesterol and quitting smoking.

12. MI (myocardial infarction) risk increases rapidly following RA diagnosis, suggesting the importance of additional mechanisms other than atherosclerosis.

13. Neither CRP nor swollen joints were predictors of heart disease progression, but joint count (number of joints affected) was.

14. A protein called NT-proBNP was shown to be a "powerful predictor" of cardiovascular risk in RA patients taking certain NSAIDs.

15. Baseline C-reactive protein level was not associated with cardiovascular event rates in the MEDAL analysis.

16. Comprehensive cardiac magnetic resonance imaging (cMRI) detects abnormalities in RA patients with no known cardiac symptoms.

17. Internal carotid artery IMT (intima-media thickness) had a higher predictive power for the development of cardiovascular events than the common carotid artery.

18. Atherosclerosis can advance while RA symptoms are quiet.

19. Some biologics may slow the thickening of arteries.

20. Prednisone decreases inflammation, but is associated with increased plaque.

(Original article with all footnotes.)[61]

FOUR: Skin involvement

Patients may experience rashes, redness, or other skin conditions such as Raynaud's phenomenon. Raynaud's is a rare blood vessel condition that can limit blood supply to fingers and toes. Raynaud's is more common in people with RD, and like Sjögren's syndrome, can be considered an extra-articular symptom in PRD. According to Cedars-Sinai hospital, Raynaud's can also be the first sign of RD.[62]

Vitiligo is a rare skin disorder characterized by the destruction of melanin cells that leaves skin with white un-pigmented areas. It is considered to be autoimmune in origin and responds to some DMARDs used in RD. Vitiligo is more common in people with RD or other immune mediated diseases, and a diagnosis of vitiligo increases the odds of a diagnosis of RA or other autoimmune disease.[63]

Nodules are a symptom that is more distinct to RD. Rheumatoid nodules can emerge on organs such as the lungs or on a musculoskeletal component such as a tendon, or more noticeably, on the skin. The cause of rheumatoid nodules is not known. They vary greatly in size, consist of firm fibrous tissue, and sometimes resolve on their own or with disease treatment. Many believe that nodules accompany more severe disease.

Livedo reticularis (LR) is a vascular rash that creates a red lacy pattern on the skin. LR is related to vasculitis in either RD or SLE. It can be difficult to obtain a diagnosis for LR, because the symptoms can be intermittent and because doctors do not always know LR can be associated with RD.[64, 65] Many expert sources including Mayo Clinic list SLE as a possible cause, but not RD.

LR occurs when some small blood vessels are blocked or no longer feed surface tissues. Other vessels enlarge to compensate, creating a netted or "reticulated" pattern. LR can be confusing because the "same term is used to refer to a harmless pattern on the skin that is common in cold weather and a more lasting symptom related to vasculitis or other more serious conditions. One easy way to tell the difference is that LR from physiologic causes, like cold, resolve with skin warming, but LR associated with rheumatoid vasculitis is still apparent after warming.[66] The condition can also be caused as a side effect of some medications such as amantadine (for Parkinson's disease) or interferon (for melanoma)."[67]

It is impossible to detail every kind of rash that PRD have experienced, but the symptom of rashes was one of the first extra-articular features to be described historically. Rash is listed as a symptom in historic descriptions of rheumatoid disease and many modern medical sources. As I described in the Introduction, I experienced a bright red symmetrical rash, repeatedly covering both arms for several months during the onset of full-blown RD. However, I have heard accounts of differing types of rashes from patients.

In current medical literature, rash is much more commonly considered in juvenile rheumatoid arthritis (JRA). In a classic and often-cited 1986 study of "classification criteria for a diagnosis of juvenile rheumatoid arthritis," Cassidy et al. refer to the "typical JRA rash" occurring in children with systemic onset JRA.[68] Twelve years later, Lawrence et al. call it the "rheumatoid rash."[69] It is a rash that comes and goes, sometimes along with a fever.

This is a good example of the fact that more observation and deliberation in JRA, also called juvenile idiopathic arthritis (JIA), has resulted in creating multiple sub-classes, with more emphasis on discerning the systemic disease aspects. While many PRD report rashes, like with other systemic issues, there is no stratification of symptoms or symptom patterns in RD. This needs to be addressed in adult RD especially for the serious health threats discussed in this book. SLE patients are already divided into six "classes"[70] and rheumatologists are developing an even more elaborate classification system.[71] Asthma phenotypes are also being developed to improve individualized treatment.[72] Further, MS patients are now being classified according to disease activity and progression.[73]

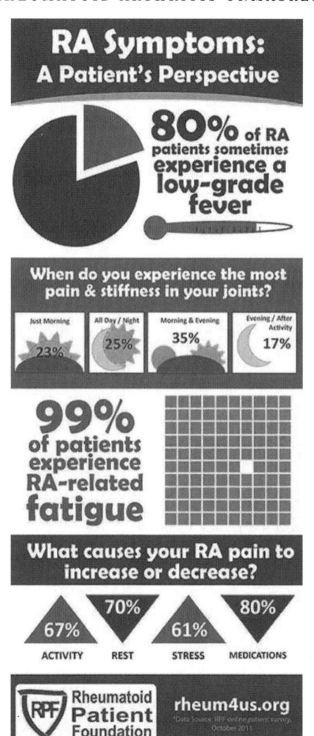

FIVE: Constitutional symptoms including fever, weight loss (cachexia), Sjögren's syndrome, and fatigue

Several constitutional symptoms of rheumatoid disease are well-documented and widely recognized including fatigue,[74] fever, and weight loss,[75] as well as "malaise, generalized stiffness, and generalized arthralgias or myalgias."[76] The symptoms are distinctive and chronic, and affect patients' daily lives: "Little attention has been paid by health professional teams to the multidimensional nature of RA-related fatigue and its wide-ranging consequences for quality of life. Unlike normal tiredness, fatigue is chronic, typically not related to overexertion and poorly relieved by rest."[77]

Some researchers have found systemic symptoms such as weight loss are evidence of more serious disease.[78] "Rheumatoid cachexia, loss of muscle mass and strength and concomitant increase in fat mass, is very common in patients with rheumatoid arthritis (RA). Despite great advances in the treatment of RA, it appears that rheumatoid cachexia persists even after joint inflammation improves. Rheumatoid cachexia may be an important risk factor for cardiovascular disease and excess mortality in RA."[79] Cachexia is linked to metabolic syndrome and was found to be associated with higher cholesterol and low-density lipoprotein, but not dietary fat intake.[80]

Loss of appetite is another common constitutional manifestation which may, along with cachexia, account for the anorexia (persistent unintended weight loss) which can be associated with RD. Various types of dietary deficiencies commonly occur with the disease, including vitamin D.[81, 82] Anemia occurs in almost one-third of PRD, increased three-fold compared to the general population[83] and has been associated with bone damage on x-ray.[84] Weakness or "flu-like" symptoms are frequently described by patients and in literature as rheumatoid symptoms; they may result from anemia, cachexia, or the "generalized arthralgias or myalgias"[85] mentioned above.

Sjögren's syndrome frequently occurs in PRD, impairing exocrine glands, causing dry eyes and mouth.[86] Sjögren's is a rheumatic diagnosis that tends to result in higher disease activity levels in RD. According to He at al., PRD with secondary Sjögren's syndrome "had more severe arthritis; a higher incidence of haematological (blood) abnormality, fever and rash; and a higher frequency of RF, ANAs and anti-SSA and anti-SSB antibodies."

Constitutional[87] manifestations frequently occur before joint symptoms,[88] and have been shown to continue despite RD treatment[89] or when obvious joint symptoms diminish.[90] They may also be associated with increased disease severity.[91] However, these commonly recognized systemic disease symptoms are not utilized in typical disease activity measures.[92] Consequently, they are not typically measured in clinical trials or in clinical practice, and frequently remain untreated. Comparatively few research studies can be found on these topics.

Risks related to infections are increased in PRD. The rate of cause of death due to infection is 9% with RA according to a compilation of literature published worldwide; this compares to a 1% rate in the general population.[93] Research has shown that both the disease and treatments can contribute to increased infection rates and increased risk of dying from infection in PRD.[94] The disease plays a role because, as described in the Chapter 1, RD is essentially an immune system disruption. As Franklin et al. describe, medications, including

DMARDs and corticosteroids also impact infection risk because they suppress immune activity. Positive rheumatoid factor has also shown to be an "independent predictor(s) of infection-related hospitalisation," indicating that disease severity impacts infection risk.

Fever is the most easily measured constitutional RD symptom that is not measured. The following is an article I wrote about fevers in RD.

The following passage was adapted from an article on rawarrior.com[95]

RHEUMATOID ARTHRITIS FEVERS

Last week, I mentioned my "rheumatoid arthritis fevers" in another post. What a surprising variety of reactions! Some said, "Me too." Others said, "Oh my, I had no idea the fever was from RA!" And others said, "What on earth do you mean by RA fever?"

What do you mean by "Rheumatoid Arthritis fever"?

When Mayo Clinic *defines* Rheumatoid Arthritis (RA), they mention fever. You also see "fever" included if you read Mayo Clinic's list of RA symptoms.[96] Fever is listed by Johns Hopkins as a symptom that precludes a "designation of complete clinical remission" in their discussion of ACR diagnostic guidelines.[97] The American College of Rheumatology website mentions fever in their explanation of RA.[98] If you read historical descriptions of RA, you will notice that fever is mentioned along with redness or rashes and crippling pain.

Typically, a rheumatoid fever is a low-grade fever. A low-grade fever is usually considered to be less than 100.4 degrees

Fahrenheit. A normal body temperature for most people is 98.6, so a low-grade fever should be a temperature between 98.7 and 100.4. However, for several years, my daily RA fever was 101.

What causes a RA fever?

- According to eMedicine, "A mildly elevated temperature is not unusual in a person with active inflammation from rheumatoid arthritis."[99]

- RA inflammation is related to cytokine activity. Fevers are related to cytokines, too.[100]

- Researchers believe that the typical fevers of systemic onset juvenile RA are related to serum levels of "the proinflammatory cytokine" IL-6.[101]

- According to an exciting article from the University of Colorado Denver, it's IL-1.[102] They diluted a form of IL-1 a million times and it still triggered lymphocytes that cause fever. In 2009, as a result of his work on this project, Dr. Dinarello won the largest award in medicine or science in the United States.

Why doesn't everyone know about RA fever?

This puzzles me. Frankly, RA is a puzzle in many ways. There is much misinformation and misleading information. Many patients know exactly what RA is, but sometimes it seems like they are the only ones. And they don't always speak freely about what daily RA is like, even to doctors, because so often they struggle to resist the mantle of hypochondriac.[103] (It is doctors and the Arthritis Foundation who have used that word, not me.)

It is typical for people with RA to have a fever. If the RA is not "controlled" or the patient has flares, there will likely be a fever as one indicator of that. So, why is this "textbook" and "typical" symptom of RA discussed so little today?

Why is it that fever, the one known typical RA symptom that is objectively measurable, is hardly measured?

Whenever I take my child to the pediatrician, the nurse takes his temperature. *However, I have never had my temperature taken at a rheumatology appointment.* Once I requested it, and the medical assistant became very frustrated because she did not know why She said, "We don't do that here."

Why not?

Isn't a fever a sign of inflammation in the body? Wouldn't it be important to use body temperature patterns as a measure of RA activity? It seems to associate more with disease activity than blood tests do.[104]

How often does your rheumatologist take your temperature? How often do you have a low-grade fever? Do you own a good digital thermometer?

(Patient discussion with over one hundred comments follows.)

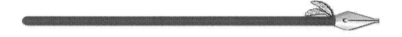

KEY POINTS

1. Some research shows RD may begin in the mouth.

2. RD affects the larynx up to 90% of the time, especially the vocal cords. Symptoms include hoarse voice or shortness of

breath.

3. Larynx involvement can be the first symptom of RD and it can be affected several ways.

4. RD can cause CV changes very early in the disease and it can involve any part of the heart, especially the left ventricle. Rheumatoid heart disease is distinct and contributes to a mortality gap. CV effects persist even if joint symptoms improve (Ch 2).

5. RD can affect the skin in several ways and can be the first sign of RD.

6. RD causes constitutional symptoms such as fever, fatigue, Sjogren's syndrome, and cachexia (loss of lean body mass). Symptoms can occur before joint symptoms and can persist even if joints improve.

Action step: Abandon expectations of RD as a "type of arthritis" that only affects joints. Patients and caregivers must treat whatever RD symptoms patients actually experience.

Quote to remember: Risks of specific CVD manifestations have been shown to exist, some already at the point of RD diagnosis. It is imperative to learn how the disease process leads to such risks. This is the crucial work of investigators who have asked: What makes PRD die prematurely, and how can it be stopped?

---

[1] Cojocaru et al. Extra-articular manifestations in rheumatoid arthritis. (See footnote Chapter 3.)

[2] Cojocaru et al. Extra-articular manifestations in rheumatoid

arthritis. (See footnote Chapter 3.)

3 Totaro MC, Cattani P, Ria F, Tolusso B, Gremese E, Fedele AL, D'Onghia S, Marchetti S, Di Sante G, Canestri S, et al. Porphyromonas gingivalis and the pathogenesis of rheumatoid arthritis: Analysis of various compartments including the synovial tissue. Arthritis Res Ther. 2013 Jun 18 [cited 2017 Mar 4];15:R66. Available from: http://arthritis-research.com/content/15/3/R66

4 Hamden AL, El-Khatib M, Dagher W, Othman I. Laryngeal involvement in rheumatoid arthritis. M.E.J. Anest. 2007 [cited 2013 Apr 20];19(2):335-346. Available from: http://www.meja.aub.edu.lb/downloads/19_2/335.pdf

5 Hamden et al. Laryngeal involvement. (See footnote Chapter 5.)

6 Hamdan et al. Laryngeal manifestations of rheumatoid arthritis. (See footnote Chapter 2.)

7 BeirithI SC, IkinoII CMY, PereiraIII IA. Laryngeal involvement in rheumatoid arthritis. Braz J Otorhinolaryngol. 2013 Apr [cited 2017 Mar 5];79(2). Available from: http://www.scielo.br/scielo.php?script=sci_arttext&pid=S1808-86942013000200017&lng=en&nrm=iso&tlng=en

8 Lofgren RH, Montgomery WW. Incidence of laryngeal involvement in rheumatoid arthritis. New Engl J Med 1962 Jul 26 [cited 2013 Apr 20]; 267:193-195. DOI: 10.1056/NEJM196207262670407

9 Bienenstock H, Ehrlich GE, Freyberg RH. Rheumatoid arthritis of the cricoarytenoid joint: A clinicopathologic study. Arthritis Rheum. 1963 Feb [cited 2013 Apr 20];6(1):48-63. DOI: 10.1002/art.1780060106

10 Bayar N, Kara SA, Keleş I, Koç C, Altinok D, Orkun S. Cricoarytenoiditis in rheumatoid arthritis: Radiologic and clinical study [abstract]. J Otolaryngol. 2003 Dec [cited 2013 Apr 20];32(6):

373-8. Available from: http://www.ncbi.nlm.nih.gov/pubmed/14967082

[11] Charlin B, Brazeau-Lamontagne L, Levesque RY, Lussier A. Cricoarytenoiditis in rheumatoid arthritis: Comparison of fibrolaryngoscopic and high resolution computerized tomographic findings [abstract]. J Otolaryngol. 1985 Dec [cited 2013 Apr 20]; 14(6):381-6. Available from: http://www.ncbi.nlm.nih.gov/pubmed/4078961

[12] Geterud A, Bake B, Berthelsen B, Bjelle A, Ejnell H. Laryngeal involvement in rheumatoid arthritis [abstract]. Acta Otolaryngol. 1991 [cited 2013 Apr 20];111(5):990-8. Available from: http://www.ncbi.nlm.nih.gov/pubmed/1759587

[13] Hamdan et al. Laryngeal manifestations of rheumatoid arthritis. (See footnote Chapter 2.)

[14] Yunt ZX. Lung disease in rheumatoid arthritis. (See footnote Chapter 2.)

[15] Bienenstock et al. Rheumatoid arthritis of the cricoarytenoid joint. (See footnote Chapter 5.)

[16] Bayar et al. Cricoarytenoiditis in rheumatoid arthritis: Radiologic and clinical study. (See footnote Chapter 5.)

[17] Bengtsson M, Bengtsson A. Cricoarytenoid arthritis — A cause of upper airway obstruction in the rheumatoid arthritis patient. Intens Care Med. 1998 Jun [cited 2013 Apr 20];24(6):643

[18] Hamdan et al. Laryngeal manifestations of rheumatoid arthritis. (See footnote Chapter 2.)

[19] Berjawi G, Uthman I, Mahfoud L, Husseini ST, Nassar J, Kotobi A, Hamdan ALH. Cricothyroid joint abnormalities in patients with rheumatoid arthritis [abstract]. J Voice. 2010 Nov [cited 2013 Apr

20];24(6):732-737. Available from: http://www.jvoice.org/article/
S0892-1997(09)00087-3/abstract

[20] Voulgari PV, Papazisi D, Bai M, Zagorianakou P, Assimakopoulos
D, Drosos AA. Laryngeal involvement in rheumatoid arthritis.
Rheumatol Int. 2005 Jun [cited 2013 Apr 20];25(5):321-5.

[21] Pinals RS. Rheumatoid arthritis presenting with laryngeal
obstruction. Brit Med J. 1966 [cited 2013 Apr 20] April 2; 1(5491):
842. Available from: http://www.ncbi.nlm.nih.gov/pmc/articles/
PMC1844320/pdf/brmedj02544-0050.pdf PMCID: PMC1844320

[22] Guerra LG, Lau KY, Marwah R. Upper airway obstruction as the
sole manifestation of rheumatoid arthritis [abstract]. J Rheumatol
[Internet]. 1992 Jun [cited 2031 Apr 20];19(6):974-6. Available from:
http://www.ncbi.nlm.nih.gov/pubmed/1404138

[23] Bertolani MF, Bergamini BM, Marotti F, Giglioli P, Venuta A.
Cricoarytenoid arthritis as an early sign of juvenile chronic arthritis
[abstract]. Clin Exp Rheumatol. 1997 Jan-Feb [cited 2013 Apr 20];
15(1):115-6. Available from: http://www.ncbi.nlm.nih.gov/pubmed/
9093786

[24] Young K. Cricoarytenoid arthritis in rheumatoid arthritis, Part 3.
Rheumatoid Arthritis Warrior [website]. 2009 Nov 11 [cited 2013
Apr 20] Available from: http://rawarrior.com/cricoarytenoid-
arthritis-in-rheumatoid-arthritis-part-3/

[25] Edelist G. Principles of anesthetic management in rheumatoid
arthritic patients. Anesth Analg. 1964 May-Jun [cited 2013 Apr 20];
43(3):227-231. Available from: http://www.anesthesia-
analgesia.org/content/43/3/227.full.pdf

[26] Voulgari et al. Laryngeal involvement in rheumatoid. (See footnote
Chapter 5.)

[27] Hamden et al. Laryngeal involvement. (See footnote Chapter 5.)

[28] Hamden et al. Laryngeal involvement. (See footnote Chapter 5.)

[29] Iacovou E, Vlastarakos PV, Nikolopoulos TP. Laryngeal involvement in connective tissue disorders. Is it important for patient management? Indian J Otolaryngol. 2014 Jan [cited 2017 Aug 1]; 66(Suppl 1):22-29. DOI:10.1007/s12070-012-0491-z

[30] Bywaters EGL. The relation between heart and joint disease including "rheumatoid heart disease" and chronic post-rheumatic arthritis. Brit Heart J. 1950 [cited 2013 Apr 20];12:101-131. Available from: http://heart.bmj.com/content/12/2/101.long

[31] Egelius N, Gohle O, Jonsson E, Wahlgren F. Cardiac changes in rheumatoid arthritis. Ann Rheum Dis. 1955 [cited 2013 Apr 20];14: 11-18. Available from: http://ard.bmj.com/content/14/1/11.long DOI: 10.1136/ard.14.1.11

[32] Handforth CP, Woodbury JFL. Cardiovascular manifestations of rheumatoid arthritis. Canad. M. A. J. 1959 Jan 15 [cited 2013 Apr 20];80:86-90. Available from: http://www.ncbi.nlm.nih.gov/pmc/articles/PMC1830563/pdf/canmedaj00797-0011.pdf

[33] Schoene RH, Risse GB. Rheumatoid heart disease. A case study with illustrations. Ohio State Med J. 1964 Apr [cited 2013 Apr 20]; 60:377-9. Title available from: http://www.ncbi.nlm.nih.gov/pubmed/14137096

[34] Kampmeier RH. Cardiac disease in rheumatoid arthritis. South Med J. 1963 May [cited 2013 Apr 20];56:563-4. Title available from: http://www.ncbi.nlm.nih.gov/pubmed/13962136

[35] Lebowitz W. The heart in rheumatoid arthritis (rheumatoid disease): A clinical and pathological study of sixty-two cases. Ann Intern Med. 1963 Jan 1 [cited 2013 Apr 20];58(1):102-123. Title and abstract available from: http://annals.org/article.aspx?

articleid=678486

[36] Kirk J, Cosh J. Rheumatoid heart disease. Ann Rheum Dis. 1969 Nov [cited 2013 Apr 20];28(6): 680–681. Available from: http://ard.bmj.com/content/28/6/680.long

[37] Rødevand E, Bathen J, Ostensen M. Rheumatoid arthritis and heart disease [abstract]. Tidsskr Nor Laegeforen. 1999 Jan 20 [cited 2013 Apr 20];119(2):223-225. Available from: http://www.ncbi.nlm.nih.gov/pubmed/10081354

[38] Boers et al. Making an impact on mortality in rheumatoid arthritis. (See footnote Chapter 3.)

[39] Centers for Disease Control and Prevention [website]. CDC heart disease facts. 2015 Aug 10 [cited 2017 Feb 26]. Available from: https://www.cdc.gov/heartdisease/facts.htm

[40] Manzi S, Wasko MCM. Inflammation-mediated rheumatic diseases and atherosclerosis. Ann Rheum Dis. 2000 [cited 2017 Mar 5]; 59:321-5. http://ard.bmj.com/content/59/5/321.full

[41] Bhatia GS, Left ventricular systolic dysfunction. (See footnote Chapter 2.)

[42] Gonzalez A, Kremers HM, Crowson CS, Nicola PJ, Davis JM, Therneau TM, Roger VL, Gabriel SE. The widening mortality gap between rheumatoid arthritis patients and the general population. Arthritis Rheum. 2007 Nov [cited 2013 Apr 21];56(11):3583–3587. Available from: http://onlinelibrary.wiley.com/doi/10.1002/art.22979/full DOI: 10.1002/art.22979.

[43] Crowson CS, Matteson EL, Roger VL, Therneau, Gabriel SE. Usefulness of risk scores to estimate the risk of cardiovascular disease in patients with rheumatoid arthritis. Am J Cardiol. 2012 Aug 1 [cited 2013 Apr 21]; 110(3):420-424. Available from: http://

www.ajconline.org/article/S0002-9149(12)01060-0/fulltext

[44] Bhatia GS, Left ventricular systolic dysfunction. (See footnote Chapter 3.)

[45] Levendoglu F, Temizhan A, Ugurlu H, Ozdemir A, Yazici M. Ventricular function abnormalities in active rheumatoid arthritis: A Doppler echocardiographic study. Rheumatol Int. 2004 May [cited 2017 Mar 5];24(3):141-146. Available from: https:// www.ncbi.nlm.nih.gov/pubmed/12819928

[46] Bharti BB, Kumar S, Kapoor A, Agarwal A, Mishra R, Sinha N. Assessment of left ventricular systolic and diastolic function in juvenile rheumatoid arthritis. J Postgrad Med. 2004 Oct-Dec[cited 2017 Mar 5];50(4):262-7. Available from: https:// tspace.library.utoronto.ca/bitstream/1807/3973/1/jp04090.pdf

[47] Bharti et al. Assessment of left ventricular systolic and diastolic function in JRA. (See footnote Chapter 5.)

[48] Kelly C, Hamilton J. What kills patients with rheumatoid arthritis? (Oxford) Rheumatology. 2007 [cited 2013 Jun 5];46 (2):183-184. Available from: http://rheumatology.oxfordjournals.org/content/ 46/2/183.full

[49] Mayo Clinic. Predicting cardiovascular disease risk for rheumatoid arthritis patients. Science Daily (website). 2007 Nov 11 [cited 2017 Jul 25]. Available from: https://www.sciencedaily.com/releases/ 2007/11/071107181025.htm

[50] Vizzardi E, Cavazzana I, Ceribelli A, Tincani A, Dei Cas L, Franceschini F. Letter: Aortic stiffness and left ventricular hypertrophy in rheumatoid arthritis: Comment on the article by Rudominer et al. Arthritis Rheum. 2009 Sep [cited 2017 Mar 12]; 60(9):2852–2853. DOI:10.1002/art.24813

[51] Södergren A, Karp K, Boman K, Eriksson C, Lundström E, Smedby

T, Söderlund L, Rantapää-Dahlqvist S, Wållberg-Jonsson S. Atherosclerosis in early rheumatoid arthritis: Very early endothelial activation and rapid progression of intima media thickness. Arthritis Res Ther. 2010 Aug 16 [cited 2013 Apr 21];12(4):158. Available from: http://arthritis-research.biomedcentral.com/articles/10.1186/ar3116 DOI: 10.1186/ar3116

[52] Myasoedova E, Davis JM, Crowson CS, Roger VL, Karon BL, Borgeson DD, Therneau TM, Matteson EL, Rodeheffer RJ, Gabriel SE. Rheumatoid arthritis is associated with left ventricular concentric remodeling: Results of a population-based cross-sectional study. Arthritis Rheum. 2013 Jul [cited 2016 Mar 4]; 65(7): 1713–1718. Available from: http://www.ncbi.nlm.nih.gov/pmc/articles/pmid/23553738/ DOI: 10.1002/art.37949

[53] Mantel Ä, Holmqvist M, Jernberg T, Wållberg-Jonsson S, Askling J. Long-term outcomes and secondary prevention after acute coronary events in patients with rheumatoid arthritis. Ann Rheum Dis. 2017 Aug 20 [cited 2017 Oct 17]. DOI: 10.1136/annrheumdis-2017-211608

[54] McInness, IB. Treatment of rheumatoid arthritis when the patient is not well, American College of Rheumatology annual scientific meeting, 2016 Nov 14 [cited 2017 Mar 4]. Available from: http://acr.peachnewmedia.com/store/seminar/seminar.php?seminar=84767

[55] Solomon DH, Peters MJL, Nurmohamed MT, Dixon W. Unresolved questions in rheumatology: Motion for debate: The data support evidence-based management recommendations for cardiovascular disease in rheumatoid arthritis. Arthritis Rheum. 2013 Jul 2 [cited 2017 Mar 12];65:1675–1683. DOI:10.1002/art.37975

[56] Mayo Clinic [website]. Cardiovascular Diseases. 2017 Jun 22 [cited 2017 Jul 3]. Available from: http://www.mayoclinic.org/departments-centers/cardiovascular-diseases/sections/specialty-

groups/orc-20122387

[57] Prasad M, Hermann J, Gabriel SE, Weyand CM, Mulvagh S, Mankad R, Oh JK, Matteson EL, Lerman A. Cardiorheumatology: Cardiac involvement in systemic rheumatic disease. Nat Rev Cardiol. 2015 Mar [cited 2017 Jul 23];12(3):168-176. Available from: https://www.ncbi.nlm.nih.gov/pmc/articles/PMC4641514

[58] National Institutes of Health [website]. Summaries for all NIH research grants are organized by year. Grants mentioned in text, in order of mention: 5R01HL123064-02, 4R01AR046849-15, 4R01AR064546-04. Estimates of Funding for Various Research, Condition, and Disease Categories. 2017 Jul 2 [cited 2017 Aug 1] Available from: https://report.nih.gov/categorical_spending.aspx

[59] Wilton KM, Matteson EL, Crowson CS. Risk of obstructive sleep apnea and its association with cardiovascular and noncardiac vascular risk in patients with rheumatoid arthritis: A population-based study. J Rheumatol. 2017 Aug [cited 2017 Sep 18]. DOI: https://doi.org/10.3899/jrheum.170460

[60] Young K. 20 Facts about rheumatoid heart disease. Rheumatoid Arthritis Warrior [website]. 2011 Apr 18 [cited 2013 Apr 21]. Available from: http://rawarrior.com/20-facts-about-rheumatoid-heart-disease/

[61] Young K. 20 Facts about rheumatoid heart disease. (See footnote Chapter 5.)

[62] Cedars-Sinai [website]. Raynaud's phenomenon. 2010 Apr 7 [cited 2017 Jul 8]. Available from: https://www.cedars-sinai.edu/Patients/Health-Conditions/Raynauds-Phenomenon.aspx

[63] Saleem K, Azim W. Association of vitiligo with other autoimmune disorders. Diabetes Case Rep. 2016 Oct 25 [cited 2017 Jul 8];1:114. Available from: https://www.omicsgroup.org/journals/association-

of-vitiligo-with-other-autoimmune-disorders-.php?aid=81738

[64] Young K. Livedo reticularis & rheumatoid arthritis: Nothing rash about It. RA Warrior [website]. 2013 Jan 15 [cited 2017 Jul 5]. Available from:http://rawarrior.com/livedo-reticularis-rheumatoid-arthritis-nothing-rash-about-it/

[65] Young K. Livedo reticularis diagnosis – She knelt next to me with a medical textbook. RA Warrior [website]. 2013 May 9 [cited 2017 Jul 5]. Available from: http://rawarrior.com/livedo-reticularis-diagnosis-she-knelt-next-to-me-with-a-medical-textbook/

[66] Gibbs MB, English JC 3rd, Zirwas MJ. Livedo reticularis: An update. J Am Acad Dermatol. 2005 Jun [cited 2017 Jul 1];52(6): 1009-19. DOI: 10.1016/j.jaad.2004.11.051

[67] Young K. Livedo reticularis & rheumatoid arthritis. (See footnote Chapter 6.)

[68] Cassidy JT, Levinson JE, Bass JC, Baum J, Brewer EJ, Fink CW, Hanson V, Jacobs JC, Masi AT, Schaller JG, et al. A study of classification criteria for a diagnosis of juvenile rheumatoid arthritis. Arthritis Rheum. 1986 Feb [cited 2017 Jul 15];29(2):274–81. Available from: http://onlinelibrary.wiley.com/doi/10.1002/art. 1780290216/full

[69] Lawrence et al. Estimates of the prevalence of arthritis and selected musculoskeletal disorders. (See footnote Chapter 3.)

[70] Wright B, Bharadwaj S. Systemic lupus erythematosus. Cleveland Clinic Center for Continuing Education [website]. 2010 Aug [cited 2015 Jul 25]. Available from: http://www.clevelandclinicmeded.com/medicalpubs/diseasemanagement/rheumatology/systemic-lupus-erythematosus/

[71] Sullivan MG. New classification system for systemic lupus erythematosus moves forward. Rheumatology News [website], 2017

Jul 20 [cited 2017 Jul 25]. Available from: http://www.mdedge.com/rheumatologynews/article/142941/lupus-connective-tissue-diseases/new-classification-system-systemic

[72] Corren J. Asthma phenotypes and endotypes: An evolving paradigm for classification. Discovery Medicine [website]. 2013 Apr 26 [cited 2017 Jul 25]. Available from: http://www.discoverymedicine.com/Jonathan-Corren/2013/04/26/asthma-phenotypes-and-endotypes-an-evolving-paradigm-for-classification/

[73] National Multiple Sclerosis Society [website]. Types of MS. 2016 Mar 3 [cited 2017 Jul 15]. Available from: http://www.nationalmssociety.org/What-is-MS/Types-of-MS

[74] Mayoux-Benhamou MA. Fatigue and rheumatoid arthritis. Annales de Réadaptation et de Médecine Physique. 2006 Jul [cited 2013 May 4];49(6):385–388. Available from: http://www.sciencedirect.com/science/article/pii/S0168605406001292

[75] Centers for Disease Control and Prevention. Rheumatoid arthritis. (See footnote Chapter 3.)

[76] Wilke WS. Rheumatoid arthritis. Cleveland Clinic [website]. 2010 Aug 10 [cited 2013 May 4]. Available from: http://www.clevelandclinicmeded.com/medicalpubs/diseasemanagement/rheumatology/rheumatoid-arthritis/

[77] Mayoux-Benhamou MA. Fatigue and rheumatoid arthritis. (See footnote Chapter 5.)

[78] Fleming A, Dodman S, et al. Extra-articular features in early rheumatoid disease. (See footnote in Chapter 1.)

[79] Roubenoff R. Rheumatoid cachexia: A complication of rheumatoid arthritis moves into the 21st century. Arthritis Res Ther. 2009 [cited 2013 May 5];11:108. Available from: http://arthritis-

research.biomedcentral.com/articles/10.1186/ar2658 DOI:10.1186/ar2658

[80] Elkan A, Håkansson N, Frostegård J, Cederholm T, Hafström I. Rheumatoid cachexia is associated with dyslipidemia and low levels of atheroprotective natural antibodies against phosphorylcholine but not with dietary fat in patients with rheumatoid arthritis: A cross-sectional study. Arthritis Res Ther. 2009 [cited 2013 May 5];11:R37. Available from: http://arthritis-research.com/content/11/2/R37

[81] Collins R, Dunn TL, Walthaw J, Harrell P, Alarcon GS. Malnutrition in rheumatoid arthritis [abstract]. Clin Rheumatol. 1987 Sep [cited 2013 May 7];6(3):391-8. Available from: http://www.ncbi.nlm.nih.gov/pubmed/3442963

[82] Attar SM. Vitamin D deficiency in rheumatoid arthritis. Prevalence and association with disease activity in Western Saudi Arabia. Saudi Medical Journal. 2012 May [cited 2013 May 7];33(5):520-5. Available from: http://www.ncbi.nlm.nih.gov/pubmed/22588813

[83] Wolfe F, Michaud K. Anemia and renal function in patients with rheumatoid arthritis. J Rheumatol. 2006 [cited 2013 May 5];33(8):1516-1522. Available from: http://jrheum.org/content/33/8/1516.abstract

[84] Möller B, Everts-Graber J, Florentinus S, Li Y, Kupper H, Finckh A. Low hemoglobin predicts radiographic damage progression in early rheumatoid arthritis – Secondary analysis from a phase iii trial. Arthritis Care Res. Accepted manuscript, 2017 Sep 17 [cited 2017 Sep 29]. DOI:10.1002/acr.23427

[85] Wilke WS. Rheumatoid arthritis. (See footnote Chapter 4.)

[86] He J, Yan Ding Y, Feng M, Guo J, Xiaolin Sun, Zhao J, Yu D, Li Z. Characteristics of Sjögren's syndrome in rheumatoid arthritis. (Oxford) Rheumatology. 2013 Feb [cited 2013 May 5]. Available from: http://rheumatology.oxfordjournals.org/content/early/

2013/02/04/rheumatology.kes374.full

[87] Delaleu N, Immervoll H, Cornelius J, Jonsson R. Biomarker profiles in serum and saliva of experimental Sjögren's syndrome: Associations with specific autoimmune manifestations. Arthritis Res Ther. 2008 [cited 2013 May 5];10(1):R22. Available from: http://arthritis-research.com/content/10/1/R22

[88] Wilke WS. Rheumatoid arthritis. (See footnote Chapter 5.)

[89] van Hoogmoed D, Fransen J, Repping-Wuts H, Spee L, Bleijenberg G, van Riel PL. The effect of anti-TNF-α vs. DMARDs on fatigue in rheumatoid arthritis patients [abstract]. Scand J Rheumatol. 2013 [cited 2013 May 5];42(1):15-9. Available from: http://www.ncbi.nlm.nih.gov/pubmed/22992002 DOI: 10.3109/03009742.2012.709878

[90] He et al. Characteristics of Sjögren's syndrome. (See footnote Chapter 5.)

[91] He et al. Characteristics of Sjögren's syndrome. (See footnote Chapter 5.)

[92] Anderson J, Caplan L, Yazdany J, Robbins ML, Neogi T, Michaud K, Saag KG, O'Dell JR, Kazi S. Rheumatoid arthritis disease activity measures: American College of Rheumatology recommendations for use in clinical practice. Arthritis Care Res. 2012 [cited 2013 May 5]; 64: 640–647. Available from: http://onlinelibrary.wiley.com/doi/10.1002/acr.21649/full DOI: 10.1002/acr.21649

[93] Boers et al. Making an impact on mortality in rheumatoid arthritis. (See footnote Chapter 3.)

[94] Franklin J, Lunt M, Bunn D, Symmons D, Silman A. Risk and predictors of infection leading to hospitalisation in a large primary-care derived cohort of inflammatory polyarthritis. Ann Rheum Dis. 2006 Sep 19 [cited 2017 Mar 24];66(3):308-12. Available from:

https://www.ncbi.nlm.nih.gov/pmc/articles/PMC1856002/

95 Young K. Rheumatoid arthritis fevers. Rheumatoid Arthritis Warrior [website]. 2010 Sep 10 [cited 2013 May 4]. Available from: http://rawarrior.com/rheumatoid-arthritis-fevers/

96 Mayo Clinic [website]. Rheumatoid arthritis symptoms and causes. 2016 Mar 18 [cited 2016 Dec 9]. Available from:

http://www.mayoclinic.org/diseases-conditions/rheumatoid-arthritis/symptoms-causes/dxc-20197390

97 Johns Hopkins Arthritis Center [website]. ACR diagnostic guidelines. 2017 Aug 16 [cited 2017 Aug 16]. Available from:

https://www.hopkinsarthritis.org/physician-corner/education/arthritis-education-diagnostic-guidelines/

98 American College of Rheumatology [website]. Rheumatoid arthritis. 2011 Dec 23 [cited 2016 Dec 9]. Available from: http://www.rheumatology.org/I-Am-A/Patient-Caregiver/Diseases-Conditions/Rheumatoid-Arthritis

99 Emedicine Health [website]. Arthritis. 2016 Nov 23 [cited 2016 Dec 9]. Available from: http://www.emedicinehealth.com/arthritis/page10_em.htm

100 Leon LR. Cytokine regulation of fever. J Appl Physiol. 2002 Jun 1 [cited 2016 Dec 9]92(6);2648-2655. Available from: http://jap.physiology.org/content/92/6/2648.abstract

101 Eberhard BA, Ilowite NT. Response of systemic onset juvenile rheumatoid arthritis to etanercept: Is the glass half full or half empty? J Rheumatol. 2005 May [citd 2016 Dec 9]. Availalble from: http://www.jrheum.com/subscribers/05/05/763.html

102 Immune system pioneers share America's largest prize in medicine. University of Colorado news release [website]. 2009 Apr

24 [cited 2016 Dec 9]. Available from: http://
www.cuanschutztoday.org/professordinarelloshares/

[103] Young K. Rheumatoid arthritis pain in the twilight zone.
Rheumatoid Arthritis Warrior [website]. 2010 Feb 10 [cited 2016 Dec
9]. Available from: http://rawarrior.com/rheumatoid-arthritis-pain-
in-the-twilight-zone/

[104] Young K. Rheumatoid factor test: Should we rely on rheumatoid
factor levels? Rheumatoid Arthritis Warrior [website]. 2010 Mar 23
[cited 2016 Dec 9]. Available from: http://rawarrior.com/
rheumatoid-factor-test-should-we-rely-on-rheumatoid-factor-levels/

CHAPTER SIX
A GROWING LIST OF DANGERS: EVEN MORE EVIDENCE

Even more evidence for rheumatoid disease

Five more ways RD increases morbidity and mortality

This chapter will describe more extra-articular features of RD and present more evidence that joint inflammation (arthritis) is only one symptom of RD. For most of these topics, the facts have unfolded over several decades as increased morbidity and mortality in RD was recognized and investigated. While the conditions on this list are not the only dangers caused by RD, I hope this list will inspire both clinicians and investigators to look further at ways to address these dangers in order to improve the health of people living with RD.

We now resume our list of 10 Dangers of Rheumatoid Disease:

SIX: Rheumatoid vasculitis and blood vessel disease

Vasculitis is the inflammation of blood vessels, causing the vessel walls to become thicker, narrowing the vessel diameter, and reducing blood flow to body tissues.[1] Rheumatoid vasculitis (RV) is the occurrence of vasculitis as a result of rheumatoid disease. Blood vessels in any organ of the body can be involved, but skin is most commonly affected. Capillaries have increased permeability in RD, and especially in RV.[2]

RV presentation is extremely heterogeneous. Patients may experience visible signs from mild to severe including cutaneous ulcers, rashes, and gangrene, or critical constitutional symptoms. "RV has a predilection for the skin and may result in peripheral gangrene and deep cutaneous ulcers that tend to occur in unusual locations."[3]

Although RV is known to be a painful condition, pain was not mentioned in at least two-dozen articles that were consulted for this section, comprised of clinical research studies, websites for advocacy organizations, and well-respected medical centers. The Cleveland Clinic rheumatoid vasculitis section does affirm that RV symptoms can be painful.[4] Careful monitoring and treatment of symptoms—including pain—is necessary in case the condition becomes severe.

Incidence of RV is debated, and some say it is infrequent: "The active vasculitis associated with rheumatoid disease occurs in about 1% of this patient population."[5] However, mortality is increased with RV.[6, 7] The cause is not known, and according to the Vasculitis Foundation, there is no explicit definition of RV.[8] Sometimes other serious manifestations of RD are actually related to RV, such as ischemic bowel disease, interstitial lung disease, CVD, or neuropathy. In people with rheumatoid disease (PRD), vasculitis may be limited to a small part of an organ, such as with nailfold lesions, episcleritis, pericarditis, or pleuritis; therefore it does not prompt a systemic diagnosis of RV.[9]

A 2010 study described current opinion on RV: *"Clinical reports have estimated the prevalence of RA vasculitis at less than 1% to 5%, whereas autopsy studies have reported 15% to 31%."*[10] Such discrepancies between autopsy and clinical diagnoses are common with many aspects of RD, but even if incidence is rare, identifying RV and knowing how to treat it is critical for those patients. "The morbidity and mortality of rheumatoid vasculitis are substantial. Studies have shown that the 5-year mortality rate is 30% to 50%, with even higher rates of morbidity related to disease complications or vasculitis treatment-related toxicity." If skin symptoms are present, Bartels et al. say that "a careful search for other systemic manifestations is necessary to characterize the severity of the vasculitis presentation."

A 2016 case study of RV demonstrated RV as an initial symptom of RD. The authors found few other such cases described in the literature: "In the literature, three case reports describe vasculitis preceding or occurring early in the course of rheumatoid disease."[11] Their report challenges the long-held view that RV only occurs in long-standing RD or that systemic disease features do not predate articular symptoms.

Thrombosis (clotting of the blood) is another blood vessel threat for PRD: "Having rheumatoid arthritis tripled the risk for developing deep vein thrombosis and doubled the risk for pulmonary embolism in an analysis of data on 146,190 Taiwan residents."[12] Venous thromboembolism (obstruction of a blood vessel by a blood clot) is a serous related risk: "In general, venous thromboembolism leads to death within 30 days in 11%-30% of patients, previous data show." The *Rheumatology News* article cites other populations in which a two to three times greater risk of developing deep vein thrombosis has been seen.

Similarly, a U.S. study examined thrombosis risk using insurance claims for about 100,000 patients: "In conclusion, our results showed an increased risk of incident VTE (venous thromboembolism), both DVT (deep vein thrombosis) and PE (pulmonary embolism), for RA patients compared with non-RA patients."[13] For PRD, the hospitalization rate for these diagnoses was increased two to three fold compared with age and gender matched non-RA patients. The authors point out that the link between RA and venous thromboembolism is not yet understood, suggesting several possible causes including inflammatory cytokines that can lead to endothelial dysfunction.

> "RA IS A COMMON DISORDER WITH A MYRIAD OF PULMONARY MANIFESTATIONS."
>
> 2015, YUNT & SOLOMON

(Footnote.)[14]

SEVEN: Lung involvement

In a similar manner to cardiovascular disease, there is a history of gradual recognition of lung manifestations of RD: their relevance, prevalence, and how early they occur in the disease process.

Gradual recognition of lung disease in RD

In 1948, case studies of PRD documented "common features in what appears to have been the development of lung lesions during the early active phase of the joint process."[15] The authors underscore the work of other investigators who had demonstrated serious extra-articular disease manifestations. "Three cases of joint and lung lesions are recorded, and it is suggested that they are among the clinical manifestations of 'rheumatoid disease.'"

In 1964, evidence in autopsies confirmed the existence of lung disease in PRD, yet did not uncover proof of its rate of occurrence.[16] Talbott and Calkins wrote: "Clinicians interested in rheumatic diseases have been impressed with what appears to be a high incidence of pulmonary complaints in patients with rheumatoid arthritis. Intensive clinical and pathological study of selected patients has strengthened the concept that the rheumatoid process involves the lung or pleura in certain cases." However, they concluded that further study is needed to establish whether lung disease is actually part of the rheumatoid disease process: "It would appear that this study offers no support for the inclusion of pulmonary involvement among the constitutional manifestations of rheumatoid arthritis. On the other hand, this study is based on a small sample. While it suggests that pulmonary involvement is not a frequent manifestation of the rheumatoid process, it by no means excludes the possibility that such manifestations might be noted in the occasional patient."

Another article of the same title, *Pulmonary Involvement in Rheumatoid Arthritis*, appearing sixteen years later in 1980, summed up the developments of the previous decades. Cervantes-Perez et al. noted that pulmonary effects in RD were still a controversial subject "that requires further and more accurate investigation."[17] They explain, "pleural effusion and pleuropulmonary nodules are now considered manifestations of the widespread nature of the rheumatoid process." They note that while some remain unconvinced, "Others, on the contrary, consider the pulmonary involvement an important part of the rheumatoid disease."

Cervantes et al. describe their dramatic findings of lung biopsies: They found "Eighty percent of the RA patients had interstitial involvement, whereas 36% of control group 1 (patients with pulmonary diseases other than immunologic processes) and 16% of control group 2 (patients who died in the same period of diseases other than respiratory causes) showed evidence of it." They also found "Vascular involvement" in 76%

of the RA patients, but in only 16% and 12% in the two control groups.

Significantly, they found no correlation between the clinical appearance of joints and degree of pulmonary involvement.

Furthermore, standard examinations often did not detect lung involvement: "In agreement with former observations, our results also indicate that chest roentgenogram (x-ray) and ventilatory tests have a low diagnostic accuracy in the early detection of pulmonary involvement in RA. In addition, serological findings, including titers of RF, seem to be of little value in the clinical investigation of the pulmonary disease."[18] Yet lung disease among PRD was shown to be a distinctive and common feature of rheumatoid disease: "In summary, the pulmonary affection in the present series was a common feature showing definite histopathological patterns and very particular clinical features. Accordingly, we think that pulmonary involvement is an important part of the systemic affection of RA. Thus, it must always be investigated." The study was conducted in a hospital setting during the 1970's when people in the U.S. still sought care for moderate to severe RD at a hospital.

In 1995, a third article of the same title reviewed literature related to the topic, describing numerous specific pulmonary manifestations. Anaya et al. described distinctions between pulmonary disease caused by RD and that related to other disorders. They determined: "It is important to emphasize the systemic nature of the disease, which affects the lungs, heart, and vascular endothelium and poses a high risk for infection."[19]

Harvard's Brigham and Women's Hospital in Boston, Massachusetts has also examined lung-related mortality in rheumatoid disease using data from the large Nurses' Health

Study. Speaking for his group, Dr. Jeffrey Sparks commented, "Respiratory disease is an underappreciated cause of death in rheumatoid arthritis. This study highlights the need to recognize and address complications of rheumatoid arthritis associated with early mortality, especially respiratory disease and cardiovascular disease."[20]

Interstitial lung disease

In 1997, Gabbay et al. observed lung abnormalities consistent with interstitial lung disease (ILD) in 58% of people with "recent onset rheumatoid arthritis."[21] Thirty-six PRD with joint disease duration of an average of 13 months were studied. They determined ILD in early RA to occur frequently: 14% showed clinically significant ILD; 44% showed abnormalities compatible with ILD (although without clinically significant symptoms); and 42% showed no abnormalities consistent with ILD.

By 2009, pulmonologists recommended a protocol for the management of pulmonary risk in PRD:[22]

> 1. "All patients with RA should undergo annual screening for ILD. The clinician should evaluate for the presence of cough, dyspnea, and crackles on pulmonary auscultation. In addition, clubbing is highly suggestive of pulmonary involvement."
> 2. "A chest radiograph should be obtained at the time RA is diagnosed, then at intervals (e.g., every other year) thereafter. In patients with longstanding RA (> 10 years), an annual chest radiograph should be considered. The loss of lung volumes or interstitial markings should prompt additional evaluation."
> 3. When ILD is suspected after the above steps, they outlined procedures for the use of pulmonary function

tests (PFT) and high-resolution CT (HRCT).

Researchers at Mayo Clinic have determined that the lifetime risk of developing ILD is 7.7% for PRD and 0.9% for people without RD (about eight and a half times higher with RD).[23] They attribute inconsistencies in estimates of occurrence of ILD to the "plethora of definitions and means of detection employed to diagnose ILD and its analog." According to Mayo Clinic estimates, about one in ten PRD will be diagnosed with ILD over the lifetime of having their disease, a risk significantly higher than the general population. They admit certain limitations of their study may have underestimated risk of ILD in RA.

Other important findings concerned mortality and ILD: "The importance of identifying patients with RA who are at risk of ILD progression becomes evident when assessing the significantly higher mortality rates among these patients in our cohort. The risk of death almost tripled for RA patients with ILD, even after adjusting for age, smoking, and sex. Our findings did not confirm those of previous studies, which suggested a lower mortality among patients with RA-associated ILD versus patients with idiopathic ILD. This discrepancy may be explained in part by our population-based approach, which allowed us to more completely observe the full spectrum of disease." An update of this population-based study, published in 2017, reported a 5-year survival rate of 59.7%.[24]

Yunt and Solomon found: "The available studies indicate that patients with RA-ILD have a 3-fold increased risk of death relative to those without ILD. In addition, although overall mortality from RA seems to be decreasing, mortality from RA-ILD seems to be increasing, particularly in women and in older age groups."[25] They raise the issue of inadequate data to "confidently characterize prognosis and mortality" of people with rheumatoid-related ILD (RA-ILD). Discrepancies in incidence data are a frequent problem in RD, as mentioned above. **More investigations are needed in which an entire population of patients are screened for particular aspects of RD.** The following study by Zhang et al. used that model.

Zhang et al. investigated ILD in 550 Chinese PRD using high-resolution computed tomography (HRCT).[26] They found the incidence of "of RA-ILD was 43.1%," with most ILD occurring within two years of RA diagnosis. They determined: "ILD is often seen in the early and active stages of RA," and "the faster disease progression, (and) the worse prognosis."

Zhang et al. addressed drastic variances in RA-ILD incidence rates reported in many studies, ranging from 3.7% to 80%. They maintain that HRCT provides a sensitive approach to identify lung abnormalities at an early stage, and therefore every patient in their study underwent HRCT, regardless of whether they were symptomatic. They found "59% of patients with RA-ILD were asymptomatic," with lung disease that could have been missed if HRCT were not used in every patient studied.

In fact, Zhang et al. point out repeatedly that overt symptoms may not be present in early RA-ILD, and "(P)atients with RA-ILD have a poor prognosis." "Therefore RA patients should have a lung HRCT at the time of diagnosis, especially the males." Furthermore, they recommend all PRD be screened using a diffusing capacity for carbon monoxide (DLCO) test of pulmonary function because DLCO can detect function changes at an early stage, even when HRCT does not show lung abnormality. "Therefore, RA patients without respiratory symptoms and with normal lung HRCT should also complete the lung function tests to detect early lung damage."

Obstructive lung disease

Obstructive lung disease (OLD) is a category of lung diseases characterized by airway obstruction. Via the Rochester Epidemiology Project, Mayo Clinic investigators found OLD to be more common in PRD than in the general population and that OLD contributes to the excess mortality of PRD. Case studies they observed "suggested that bronchiectasis and constrictive bronchiolitis may represent distinct extraarticular manifestations of RA."[27] Confounding factors such as smoking were analyzed. Even when limiting their "analysis to nonsmokers, pulmonary obstruction was still twice as likely among RA patients when compared to non-RA subjects." Compared to OLD patients without rheumatoid disease, a "high proportion of pulmonary death diagnoses among RA patients with OLD (48%) is pointing toward a causal relationship between obstructive pulmonary disease and premature death in RA patients." According to Yunt's findings, bronchiectasis occurs in 16% to 58% of PRD. "Most cases are not clinically significant but, when present, symptoms include cough and sputum production. Treatment of these patients with a biologic agent has been reported as an independent risk factor for lower respiratory tract infection."[28]

It is urgent that rheumatologists and other physicians become aware of risks associated with lung disease in their patients with RD. While ILD and OLD may be more common, the following is a partial list of other lung manifestations associated with RD encountered in medical literature while researching this chapter: rheumatoid pleurisy, rheumatoid pleural effusion, rheumatoid bronchiolitis, fibrobullous disease, fibrosing alveolitis, parenchymal nodules, airway obstruction, and vasculitis. It has been 37 years since Cervantes-Perez et al.

demonstrated that pulmonary involvement is a significant aspect of extra-articular disease in RD and recommended that "it must always be investigated."[29] Yet PRD are not routinely screened for lung abnormalities and most medical sources still assert that RD lung involvement is rare and limited to late-stage disease.

Like other non-joint RD symptoms, lung involvement may be the first symptom of RD to present: "in some instances lung involvement is the first manifestation of RA and is the most aggressive feature of the disease. Clinicians should therefore remain alert to the possibility of lung disease in all patients with RA."[30] Yunt and Solomon recommend that clinicians be alert to symptoms such as a new cough, pointing out that symptoms may seem less remarkable in "patients with exercise-limiting joint disease." They suggest that initial pulmonary function tests "include components of lung volume, airflow with bronchodilator challenge, and DLCO measurements" as well as HRCT and oxygen tests both at rest and after activity.

EIGHT: Kidney disease in rheumatoid disease

A 1987 study of 132 autopsies of people with rheumatoid disease found the most common involvement was hardening of the small blood vessels in the kidneys or nephrosclerosis: "Necropsy findings included nephrosclerosis (90%), systemic vasculitis (14%) with kidney involvement in 8%, amyloidosis (11%), membranous glomerulopathy (8%), and focal glomerular disease (8%). Association with clinical data suggests that both rheumatoid and non-rheumatoid disease may play a part in the cause of these abnormalities."[31] The more difficult task is to determine the role that RD plays in these diagnoses. Boers et al. did not propose the nature of the relationship between RD and kidney disease. However, they note that

"(S)everal necropsy and biopsy studies have shown non-specific kidney changes, which were ascribed to RA."

Boers et al. maintain that their research "contradicts the assumption that renal involvement is rare in patients with this complication (vasculitis)."[32] And they suggest that these renal diagnoses should be investigated in PRD when renal abnormalities develop, especially in PRD with many extra-articular features. Their conclusion is unexpected when many sources deny the possibility of renal involvement: "In summary, our study confirms the view that the kidney is frequently damaged in the course of a lifetime with RA. The scope of renal disease in RA encompasses well known entities such as amyloidosis, vasculitis, and membranous glomerulopathy, but may be wider and include other forms of glomerulopathy and benign nephrosclerosis. The associations between renal abnormalities and clinical data suggest that RA contributes to the renal damage caused by concomitant disease."

More recently in 2004, the attributed cause of death in RA was found to be related to renal disease in 8% of cases in a large U.S population study, versus 1% in the general population.[33] A 2011 review investigated the relationship between kidney disease and rheumatic disease.[34] Again despite lack of specific evidence of whether or how RD may lead to renal disease, Anders and Vielhauer found kidney-related mortality was increased in PRD: "Regardless of the etiology, concurrent renal disease is a predictor of mortality in RA patients."

A 2014 Mayo Clinic study of 813 PRD and 813 age, gender, and BMI matched "non-RA individuals" found PRD more likely to develop reduced kidney function.[35] Hickson et al. determined that "reduced kidney function is common in patients with RA and increases in prevalence over time." Kidney disease also impacted by the CV health of PRD: "The presence of RA disease in individuals with reduced kidney function may lead to an increase in morbidity from CVD development, primarily in those with advanced kidney disease." Mortality risk was increased with RD, associated with higher estimated glomerular filtration rate (eGFR), a measure of kidney function: "During follow-up, 392 patients (RA, 229; non-RA, 163) died."

NINE: Eye involvement

Experts have said that the disease can affect any part of the body.[36] The eyes are frequently sites of inflammation, as described by a Cleveland Clinic physician: "Ocular manifestations of RA are diverse and range from mild, asymptomatic findings to aggressive, vision-threatening disease. RA is often associated with secondary Sjögren's syndrome or *keratoconjunctivitis sicca*, which can manifest with eye dryness, foreign-body sensation in the eye, or photophobia (extreme sensitivity to light). Chronic inflammation, resulting in perturbation of the intraocular anatomy, can lead to glaucoma."[37] (For more on Sjögren's syndrome, see also Chapter 5 "Constitutional symptoms.")

Both scleritis and episcleritis are also associated with RD. Scleritis may be associated with severe corneal inflammation, leading to a corneal melt, or with *scleromalacia perforans*. The Mayo Clinic story of Sandy Blue's scleritis discussed in Chapter 4 ("THREE: Improved diagnosis and increased remissions") is an example of eye involvement preceding obvious joint symptoms in RD.

A cross-sectional study of patents from six countries found eye involvement in about one-fourth of PRD.[38] They notably observed that eye manifestations in RD are related to "immune alterations" like the development of antibodies. A review of current literature on inflammatory eye disease indicates that extra-articular RD includes eye symptoms, which can—as in Sandy Blue's case—be the first signs of the disease.[39] "These inflammatory ophthalmological conditions include episcleritis, scleritis and peripheral ulcerative keratitis (PUK). RA is the leading cause of necrotizing scleritis and of PUK, which are the two most severe ocular conditions associated with the disease. These conditions can rapidly threaten ocular prognosis and are associated with excess mortality in patients with RA owing to their association with systemic vasculitis." The authors propose a decision tree to aid in treatment decisions in PRD with eye involvement.

> "RHEUMATOID ARTHRITIS (RA) IS OFTEN CHARACTERIZED BY THE BURDEN OF SWOLLEN JOINTS, PAIN, AND DECREASED PHYSICAL FUNCTION, BUT LESS UNDERSTOOD ARE THE MANY MANIFESTATIONS OF ADDITIONAL HEALTH CONDITIONS THAT ARE ASSOCIATED WITH RA AND ITS TREATMENTS... THE CHRONIC, DEBILITATING, AUTOIMMUNE NATURE OF RA AFFECTS THE PATIENT DIRECTLY OR INDIRECTLY IN ALMOST ALL ORGAN SYSTEMS..."
>
> 2007, MICHAUD & WOLFE

(Footnote.)[40]

TEN: RD effects on other organs

The spleen and other organs can also become involved in RD, but research is more limited. Here is a brief summary of how some are involved.

Felty's syndrome is one consequence of long-standing RD. It is diagnosed in PRD with a swollen spleen and low white blood count. Felty's syndrome is more common in older and female PRD. It can result in increased infections, a swollen liver, or other constitutional symptoms like fever, fatigue, and unintentional weight loss. Patients with Felty's may also have more infections.

Lymph nodes are small organs of the lymph system, present throughout the body. They are part of the adaptive immune system and involved in the activation of B and T cells. Lymph nodes can become swollen due to infections and viruses, and also from RD. Mayo Clinic and Medline Plus both list RA as a cause of swollen lymph nodes, or lymphadenopathy.[41, 42]

Lymph nodes have long been acknowledged to be affected by RD. In 1952, Motulsky et al. reported that swollen lymph nodes are actually a result of systemic disease involvement, rejecting older theories that the tiny glands were bogged down by drainage from swollen joints: "Systemic involvement of lymphoid tissue is a well-recognized feature of rheumatoid arthritis. Among patients with rheumatoid arthritis, 50 to 75% may be found to have palpable lymph nodes."[43] A more recent report found enlarged lymph nodes in 82% of PRD with active disease.[44]

Neuropathy is dysfunction of peripheral nerves often causing numbness, weakness, or pain that is considered stabbing, burning, or tingling. Several different illnesses or conditions can damage nerves, but in RD, swelling may physically compress adjacent nerves causing peripheral neuropathies. Commonly neuropathy affects the hands and feet, and can lead to injury or infection in extreme cases. Carpal tunnel syndrome is actually a localized neuropathy of the hands. When this occurs in the feet, it is called tarsal tunnel syndrome. Different types of neuropathy can also affect arms and legs, and other parts of the body. RA is usually listed as one of the conditions that can cause neuropathy. Using nerve function tests, a Turkish study found 36% of an RA group to be affected by neuropathy, but only 6% of a control group. "As a result, we conclude that peripheral nerve involvement is one of the striking extra-articular involvements of RA, with no apparent correlation with the clinical parameters" (joint swelling).[45]

The brain is an organ that has been little studied with regard to effects of RD. Recent examination by transcranial Doppler ultrasound demonstrated that arteries to the brain, including the middle cerebral artery and basilar artery, have reduced blood flow and increased plaque in RD.[46] Olah et al. conducted a thorough investigation of blood flow to the brain and its relationship to known significant arterial problems in RD. (See Chapter 5 for more on cardiovascular disease in RD.) Olah et al. also examined the response of brain blood flow to circumstances like brief hyperventilation or breath holding. Circulatory reserve capacity was found to be impaired in RD and correlated with other rheumatoid disease activity.

Blood flow in the brain is measured by ultrasound through temporal acoustic windows (TAWs), which are either foramina (normal openings in bone) or areas of thinner bone. While 8–20% of the healthy population may have inadequate TAWs, the authors found "TAW failure was significantly more common among patients with RA" (specific data published in a separate paper).[47]

Examination by MRI showed brain lesions to also be more common in PRD. Olah et al. found 39% of patients had "at least one vascular lesion in the right and left cerebral hemispheres." It is possible that any or all of these findings may be linked to the already established increased risk of stroke in PRD. Furthermore, abnormal blood flow to the brain could potentially affect other brain-related symptoms in RD such as fatigue, malaise, brain fog, or depression.

The liver is involved in metabolism of food, filtration of toxins, and production of proteins necessary for blood clotting and other functions. The liver actually performs over "500 roles" in the body.[48] RD can cause several liver abnormalities, including rheumatoid vasculitis (RV). Like heart, lung, and other organ involvement in RD, statistics on liver incidence vary greatly due to varying criteria and assessment methods. In only a few cases have investigators screened whole populations of patients with highly sensitive methods. As Yunt points out (with regard to lung studies), "wide variation reflects differences in study design, study populations, and the way that lung disease in RA is defined."[49]

In 1976, Fleming et al. found liver swelling, or hepatomegaly, in "21% overall" of their patients with RD.[50] A 2004 review of liver symptoms in rheumatic diseases quotes studies finding only 6% of PRD have abnormal liver function tests, but noted one study that found abnormal liver cells in 65% of patents and another that found 74% had "nonspecific reactive changes."[51] In a review of 62 articles on liver disease in patients with rheumatic diseases, Selmi et al. point out that "liver is often overlooked as a target organ."[52] And they acknowledge that "liver injury is not generally recognized as a significant extra-articular feature of RA." Nevertheless, studies show it may be important to clinical management of many patients: "Abnormal liver tests varying with disease activity, mainly elevated alkaline phosphatase, have been reported in 18 to 50% of patients with RA. Similarly, 65% of unselected patients with RA had abnormal liver biopsies."[53]

Romanian investigators agree: only about 6% of RD cases have documented liver effects, but liver function tests may be abnormal in 65% of people with RD.[54] Physicians must know when blood tests, biopsies, or scans are needed to confirm liver problems. While extra-articular manifestations in the liver may be rare, they are "exceptionally serious" including "intrahepatic portal hypertension without cirrhosis, amyloidosis, drug hepato-toxicity and viral interferences."[55] Although damage from medications is not a direct result of the disease, medications that are required with RD greatly increase the risk of liver injury.

Gastrointestinal (GI) problems have plagued PRD for many years due to medication side effects and damage. The GI tract is "the most frequent organ affected by adverse drug reactions in the USA."[56] And PRD are often most severely impacted because of a persistent need for anti-inflammatory medications. Gastrointestinal disease is twice as likely to be a cause of death in RD.[57] A large Mayo Clinic population-based study found that serious upper and lower GI events and GI mortality in PRD are common and can be serious.[58] Myasoedova et al. noted several types of GI events to be more frequent in PRD. Upper GI events that were significantly more common in PRD included ulcers, bleeds, and esophagitis. Increased lower GI events included infectious colitis or drug-induced colitis, particularly due to NSAID or DMARD use.

Note: It is difficult to know how much the additional GI morbidity and mortality risks in RD are a direct result of the disease, or whether they are due to persistent use of medications that cause GI injury. However, since they have historically been very significant, these GI problems have been added to this section.

Other GI involvement

Rheumatoid vasculitis, discussed above, can affect almost any organ, including the liver and GI tract in rare cases.

Inflammatory bowel disease (IBD) can cause joint inflammation that can seem similar to the arthritis of RD, but in a more limited pattern.[59] IBD can also occur in people with RD, but this comorbidity is rare according to extensive reviews of research literature.[60]

Some GI research examines possible links to the onset of RD. In 2013, a study found higher levels of an intestinal bacteria, Prevotella copri (P. copri), in people newly diagnosed with RA.[61] At the same time, there were fewer beneficial bacteria in the GI tracts these patients. Also, the P. copri found in the "newly diagnosed patients appears genetically distinct from P. copri found in healthy individuals." This and similar studies have been popularly touted as evidence that bacteria are implicated as a cause of RD. However, the authors of the study note that the increased P. copri levels may reflect either a cause or an effect of the inflammatory disease.[62, 63] New York University School of Medicine and several other centers continue to study the relationship between RD and the microbiome.

Side effects and comorbidities

The extra-articular manifestations of RD discussed in this chapter do not take into account many medication side effects or common comorbidities such as thyroid disease or rare comorbidities for which odds are increased with RD such as malignancy or opportunistic infection. Study and treatment of such conditions are vital for the improved health of PRD; however, the purpose of this chapter is to more fully recognize the scope of extra-articular RD manifestations. For some conditions, it is not yet clear which category is correct: comorbidities, complications, side effects, or extra-articular symptoms. *For a simple explanation of each category, see the Glossary and Tips chapter in the back of this book.* Also, this list of ten dangers is not an exhaustive list of all possible extra-articular manifestations of RD.

CONSEQUENCES OF FAILING TO RECOGNIZE A SERIOUS DISEASE

Misinformation is widespread

As with the heart disease of RD, the discussion of lungs progressed from queries of why PRD die earlier to whether certain serious conditions which account for increased deaths are related to the disease process. The discussion continues to areas like the identification of specific conditions occurring in PRD to the investigation of actual disease processes themselves and how to arrest them.

However, with decades of education to the contrary, some of the serious extra-articular manifestations of RD discussed in this book are frequently unmentioned, counted as rare, or otherwise minimized in media and on websites used by the public for medical information including National Institutes of Health's (NIH) National Institute of Arthritis and Musculoskeletal and Skin Diseases (NIAMS) and the Centers for Disease Control and Prevention (CDC).[64, 65, 66, 67, 68, 69, 70]

Even when these institutions acknowledge extra-articular disease manifestations, they claim they occur rarely and only in late stage disease. Alternatively extra-articular disease is blamed on lifestyle factors of PRD such as lack of exercise or medication effects.[71] Fox News, Wall Street Journal, and other news outlets have routinely published Dow Jones Newswires' coverage of news related to RD in which Jennifer Dooren has repeatedly stated as her entire description of the disease: "Rheumatoid arthritis is a chronic inflammatory disorder that usually affects small joints in the hands and feet."[72, 73, 74] This refrain is even echoed on the Medscape reference site for physicians, defining RA as an "inflammatory disorder of the small joints of the hands and feet."[75]

The mega-website About.com gets it wrong too: "The prevalence of extra-articular involvement is about 40% of patients at any time during the course of the disease"[76] (referencing a single small Italian study showing extra-articular manifestations may be less in Mediterranean peoples). As you see, popular messages are decades behind the applicable science.

Mortality: the ultimate problem with a dangerous disease

In 1986, Pincus and Callahan raised questions regarding RD mortality, its causes, and possible remedies.[77] Their editorial response to a concurrent study by Kaplan[78] attempted to grapple with some of the same issues this book confronts. Despite relying on 1977 death certificate recordings that predictably showed the rate of CVD death in RD to be in "proportions comparable to the general population," they recognized several crucial factors which may pertain to "an average shortening of survival of 3–18 years" for people with rheumatoid disease. First, they acknowledged the disadvantage of RA being considered merely a type of arthritis: "RA has generally been regarded as a 'nonfatal' disease in most patients, an impression maintained in part as musculoskeletal disease does not account for an immediate cause of death." Hence it tends to commonly not be "found on the death certificate." Pincus and Callahan explain: "a chronic disease will be listed on a death certificate… if there exists understanding of how the pathophysiology may contribute to mortality."

Further, Pincus and Callahan commented on a large 1978 survey of the U.S. population by the Social Security Administration which identified "comorbidity" as quite high in

RA: "data from the Survey indicate that individuals with arthritis report other conditions about 3-fold more frequently than the general population, not explained by age. Only about 25% of the individuals reporting 'symmetrical arthritis' reported no other health condition, while 34.4% reported hypertension and other cardiovascular disease, compared to 9.1% of the age 18-64 population not reporting any kind of arthritis." They concluded that the "striking finding may explain in part the predisposition to higher mortality in RA." Clearly, the nature of the relationship between RD, its common comorbidities, and its extra-articular features remains a matter of interest.

Pincus and Callahan suggested that future study should identify predictive markers for rheumatoid mortality as has been done with other chronic diseases. For example they mention their own previous reports of "5-year survivals of 50% or less" for PRD who are severely dysfunctional and "mortality greater than 40% over the next 5 years" in PRD who experience extra-articular disease features at diagnosis. They close with listing several physiologic factors that were then under investigation as possible activators and mediators of rheumatoid disease, placing "hope" in future understanding of the disease process. While immunological research and even the language describing immune processes and signaling has vastly advanced during the intervening decades, their conclusion remains relevant.

Insufficient statistics, but too many examples of RD-related mortality

While the topics discussed in this chapter are not the only extra-articular manifestations of RD, they have been shown to contribute to the increased mortality rate of RD, estimated to be "increased at least 2-fold" (twice the general population).[79]

The incidence of some of these manifestations is rare, and for others it is more common; however, the risk that a particular PRD will encounter one or more of them is very high. As mentioned in Chapter 3, only 8% of recent onset PRD in one study experienced no extra-articular disease manifestations and 41% experienced four or more.[80] Mortality risk seems not merely increased by specific extra-articular manifestations of RD, but from the disease itself, increasing with both the severity and duration of the disease. "Anti-CCP-positive RA was associated with substantial excess mortality among postmenopausal women."[81] Traditional risk factors did not account for increased mortality. Similarly, "(T)he increased risk among anti-CCP-positive women with RA was not explained by age, RF positivity, ANA positivity, or DMARD use."

> "PATIENTS WITH LONG-STANDING HIGH DISEASE ACTIVITY
> ARE AT SUBSTANTIALLY INCREASED RISK OF MORTALITY."
> 2013, LISTING ET AL.

(Footnote.)[82]

As discussed in Chapter 4, mortality statistics in RD are deficient. Whatever the numbers are, anecdotal evidence substantiates the gravity of the problem. While having contact with many PRD over the past nine years, I have become increasingly aware that rheumatoid-related death is a reality. We have seen several people in our patient support community die of causes related to the disease. It is a regular event. The fact that death from RD does occur ought to be reason enough to modernize the vocabulary with which we discuss the disease so that doctors and patients will have greater awareness of the dangers patients face.

In her e-book, *Death by Rheumatoid Arthritis*, Carla Veno Jones recounts the tragic death of her mother due to a compressed spinal cord, caused by rheumatoid arthritis, which her doctor described as being similar to that of Christopher Reeve.[83] Celia Veno, Carla's mother, had x-rays that confirmed the spinal damage that led to her death; but her doctors failed to detect the abnormalities. Later, Celia's new doctor delivered the bad news: "Your condition is progressive. It's as though there is a floating knife in your back. This knife consists of fragmented bone from your spine. From any small movement, this knife will cut off one or all of your bodily functions, such as your heart or your breathing. You'll die if you don't get an operation to get this repaired." When she learned that she had only a ten percent chance of surviving the surgery, Celia declined the operation. She died shortly afterward, ending her excruciating battle with RD.

One well-known person to die as a result of rheumatoid disease was television journalist Deborah Norville's mother, Merle. According to Norville, "She had a really tough case of it. She battled it for ten years, ten tough years, and she died from complications from it."[84] Deborah has spoken frequently about her mother's illness, encouraging people to seek treatment.[85]

In 2012, influential feminist poet Adrienne Rich died as a result of "complications of rheumatoid arthritis, with which she had lived most of her adult life," according to family.[86]

Conversations about stories like these are mostly limited to the community of patients and their families. But in January 2016, with reports of Eagles founder Glenn Frey's death, the discussion of RD mortality radiated to the general public. People were shocked that RD could possibly be a factor in someone's death. Then came a debate over whether RD was truly at fault for Frey's death or whether his medications were to blame.[87]

"Eagles manager Irving Azoff said that Frey's illnesses were partly caused by the medication he was taking for his rheumatoid arthritis... 'The colitis and pneumonia were side effects from all the meds,' Azoff said. 'He died from complications of ulcer and (ulcerative) colitis after being treated with drugs for his rheumatoid arthritis which he had for over 15 years.'"[88]

Whether the disease itself or the treatments led to Frey's death, it was remarkable how startled people were that there could be any connection at all between RD and someone's death.

Perception versus reality in RD mortality

A recent study of juvenile rheumatoid patients, diagnosed with Systemic Juvenile Idiopathic Arthritis (sJIA), showed lung disorders resulting from inflammation, specifically pulmonary artery hypertension (PAH), interstitial lung disease (ILD) and alveolar proteinosis (AP), "are under-recognized complications of sJIA which are frequently fatal."[89] The authors concluded, "Despite recent advances in therapy, sJIA remains a disease with significant morbidity and mortality." The data were disturbing: "Seventeen (68%) patients died at a mean of 10.2 months from pulmonary diagnosis." The children in the study suffered from severe systemic disease and were all exposed to biologic disease modifying drugs.

As we have seen, these serious disease effects occur more commonly than the medical community suspects. For this reason, doctors and nurses who care for rheumatoid patients do not know the risk for an individual patient developing particular extra-articular dangers. This makes it is more difficult for them to estimate what care is needed and provide proper treatment with the appropriate urgency.

It is an affront to these children, struggling for their lives, to say that they merely have "arthritis." The words "rheumatoid arthritis" and "juvenile arthritis" convey the impression of a condition limited to musculoskeletal symptoms, and most patients and family members can attest that they encounter that perception almost universally while they struggle with a disease that could take their lives. A disease that increases mortality deserves a label serious enough to provoke concern and curiosity, especially in the medical community where it is needed most.

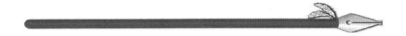

KEY POINTS

1. Rheumatoid vasculitis greatly increases mortality in PRD. It can be the first symptom of RD.

2. Rheumatoid lung disease is common and distinct. It has a long history of controversy. RD lung disease can occur in early RD without overt symptoms and can be the first symptom of RD. RD lung disease contributes to mortality.

3. PRD should have a lung HRCT scan and a DLCO breathing test at diagnosis.

4. The kidney is frequently damaged in the course of a lifetime with RA. It is 8 times more likely to be a cause of death than in people without RD.

5. Eyes can be affected by RD in several ways. Eye involvement can be the first symptom of RD.

6. Mortality is elevated for many of the extra-articular

problems of RD.

7. Misinformation about extra-articular RD is widespread, even from trusted sources and government agencies.

Action step: Do not underestimate the widespread nature of the effects of RD. Patients should be referred to whichever specialists handle each of these issues.

Quote to remember: Researchers determined: "It is important to emphasize the systemic nature of the disease, which affects the lungs, heart, and vascular endothelium and poses a high risk for infection."

---

[1] Mayo Clinic staff. Vasculitis. Mayo Clinic [website]. 2011 Oct 8 [cited 2013 Apr 22]. Available from: http://www.mayoclinic.org/diseases-conditions/vasculitis/basics/causes/con-20026049

[2] Hachulla E, Perez-Cousin M, Flipo RM, Houvenagel E, Cardon T, Catteau MH, Duquesnoy B, Devulder B. Increased capillary permeability in systemic rheumatoid vasculitis: Detection by dynamic fluorescence nailfold videomicroscopy [abstract]. Journal of Rheumatol. 1994 Jul [cited 2013 May 4];21(7):1197-202. Available from: http://www.ncbi.nlm.nih.gov/pubmed/7966057

[3] Hellmann M, Jung N, Owczarczyk K, Hallek M, Rubbert A. Successful treatment of rheumatoid vasculitis-associated cutaneous ulcers using rituximab in two patients with rheumatoid arthritis. (Oxford) Rheumatology. 2008 [cited 2013 Apr 22];47(6): 929-930. Available from: http://rheumatology.oxfordjournals.org/content/47/6/929.long

[4] Cleveland Clinic [website]. Rheumatoid vasculitis. 2011 Jun 10 [cited 2013 May 4]. Available from: http://my.clevelandclinic.org/

orthopaedics-rheumatology/diseases-conditions/hic-rheumatoid-vasculitis.aspx

[5] The Johns Hopkins Medicine [website]. Rheumatoid vasculitis. The Johns Hopkins Arthritis Center. 2005 Feb 15 [cited 2017 Mar 4]. Available from: https://www.hopkinsvasculitis.org/types-vasculitis/rheumatoid-vasculitis/

[6] Voskuyl AE, Zwinderman AH, Westedt ML, Vandenbroucke JP, Breedveld FC, Hazes JMW. The mortality of rheumatoid vasculitis compared with rheumatoid arthritis. Arthritis Rheum. 1996 Feb [cited 2013 Apr 21];39(2):266-271.

[7] Walsh, N. Death rate still high in RA vasculitis. MedPage Today [website]. 2012 May 4 [cited 2013 Apr 22]. Available from: http://www.medpagetoday.com/MeetingCoverage/BSR/32517

[8] Vasculitis Foundation [website]. Rheumatoid vasculitis. 2012 Jul 18 [cited 2013 Apr 21] Available from: [http://www.vasculitisfoundation.org/education/forms/rheumatoid-vasculitis/

[9] Voskuyl AE, Hazes JMW, Zwinderman AH, Paleolog EM, van der Meer FJM, Daha MR, Breedveld FC. Diagnostic strategy for the assessment of rheumatoid vasculitis. Ann Rheum Dis. 2003 [cited 2013 Apr 22];62:407-413. Available from: http://ard.bmj.com/content/62/5/407.long DOI:10.1136/ard.62.5.407

[10] Bartels CM, Bridges AJ. Rheumatoid vasculitis: Vanishing menace or target for new treatments? Curr Rheumatol Rep. 2010 Dec [cited 2013 May 4]; 12(6): 414–419. Available from: http://www.ncbi.nlm.nih.gov/pmc/articles/PMC2950222/

[11] Sacks S, Steuer A. Can rheumatoid vasculitis predate a diagnosis of rheumatoid arthritis? Eur J Rheumatol. 2017 Mar 4 [cited 2017 Mar 22];4(1):57-58. DOI :10.5152/eurjrheum.2017.160058

[12] Boschert S. Venous thromboembolism risk increased with rheumatoid arthritis. Rheumatology News [website]. 2013 Aug 7 [cited 2017 Mar 18]. Available from: http://www.mdedge.com/rheumatologynews/article/77004/cardiology/venous-thromboembolism-risk-increased-rheumatoid-arthritis

[13] Kim SC, Schneeweiss S, Liu J, Solomon DH. Risk of venous thromboembolism in patients with rheumatoid arthritis. Arthritis Rheum. 2013 Sep 23 [cited 2017 Mar 18];65(10):1600–1607. doi: 10.1002/acr.22039

[14] Yunt ZX. Lung disease in rheumatoid arthritis. (See footnote Chapter 2.)

[15] Ellman P. Rheumatoid disease. (See footnote Chapter 2.)

[16] Talbott JA, Calkins E. Pulmonary involvement in rheumatoid arthritis. JAMA. 1964 [cited 2013 Apr 28];189(12):911-913. DOI: 10.1001/jama.1964.03070120033008

[17] Cervantes-Perez P, Toro-Perez AH, Rodriguez-Jurado P. Pulmonary involvement in rheumatoid arthritis. JAMA. 1980 May 2 [cited 2013 Apr 28];243(17):1715-1719.

[18] Cervantes-Perez et al. Pulmonary involvement in rheumatoid arthritis. (See footnote Chapter 6.)

[19] Anaya JM, Diethelm L, Ortiz LA, Gutierrez M, Citera G, Welsh RA, Espinoza LR. Pulmonary involvement in rheumatoid arthritis. Semin Arthritis Rheu. 1995 Feb [cited 2013 Apr 27];24(4):242-254. Abstract available from: http://www.semarthritisrheumatism.com/article/S0049-0172(95)80034-4/abstract

[20] Goodman A. More respiratory deaths in rheumatoid arthritis patients. Medscape [website]. 2014 Nov 19 [cited 2017 Mar 4]. Available from: http://www.medscape.com/viewarticle/835204

[21] Gabbay E, Tarala R, Will R, Carroll G, Adler B, Cameron D, Lake FR. Interstitial lung disease in recent onset rheumatoid arthritis. Am J Respir Crit Care Med. 1997 Aug [cited 2013 Apr 28];156(2 Pt 1): 528-35. Available from: http://www.ncbi.nlm.nih.gov/pubmed/ 9279235

[22] Kim EJ, Collard HR, King TE. Rheumatoid arthritis-associated interstitial lung disease: The relevance of histopathologic and radiographic pattern. Chest. 2009 Nov [cited 2013 Apr 28];136(5): 1397–1405. Available from: http://www.ncbi.nlm.nih.gov/pmc/ articles/PMC2818853/ DOI: 10.1378/chest.09-0444 PMCID: PMC2818853

[23] Bongartz T, Nannini C, Medina-Velasquez YF, Achenbach SJ, Crowson CS, Ryu JH, Vassallo R, Gabriel SE, Matteson EL. Incidence and mortality of interstitial lung disease in rheumatoid arthritis: A population-based study. Arthritis Rheum. 2010 Jun [cited 2013 Apr 29];62(6):1583–1591. Available from: http:// onlinelibrary.wiley.com/doi/10.1002/art.27405/full DOI: 10.1002/ art.27405

[24] Zamora-Legoff JA, Krause ML, Crowson CS, Ryu JH, Matteson EL. Patterns of interstitial lung disease and mortality in rheumatoid arthritis. (Oxford) Rheumatology. 2016 Dec 3 [cited 2017 Mar 4];56 (3):344-350. DOI: 10.1093/rheumatology/kew391

[25] Yunt ZX. Lung disease in rheumatoid arthritis. (See footnote Chapter 2.)

[26] Zhang Y, Li H, Wu N, Dong X , Zheng Y. Retrospective study of the clinical characteristics and risk factors of rheumatoid arthritis-associated interstitial lung disease. Clin Rheumatol. 2017 Feb 12 [cited 2017 June25]. DOI:10.1007/s10067-017-3561-5

[27] Nannini C, Medina-Velasquez YF, Achenbach SJ, Crowson CS, Ryu, JH, Vassallo R, Gabriel SE, Matteson EL, Bongartz T. Incidence and

mortality of obstructive lung disease in rheumatoid arthritis: A population-based study. Arthritis Care Res. 2013 Jul 26 [cited 2017 Mar 4]65:1243–1250. doi:10.1002/acr.21986

[28] Yunt ZX. Lung disease in rheumatoid arthritis. (See footnote Chapter 2.)

[29] Cervantes-Perez et al. Pulmonary involvement in rheumatoid arthritis. (See footnote Chapter 6.)

[30] Yunt ZX. Lung disease in rheumatoid arthritis. (See footnote Chapter 2.)

[31] Boers M, Croonen AM, Dijkmans BA, Breedveld FC, Eulderink F, Cats A, Weening JJ. Renal findings in rheumatoid arthritis: Clinical aspects of 132 necropsies. Ann Rheum Dis. 1987 Sep 1 [cited 2017 Mar 18];46:658-663. Available from: http://ard.bmj.com/content/annrheumdis/46/9/658.full.pdf

[32] Boers et al. Renal findings in rheumatoid arthritis. (See footnote Chapter 6.)

[33] Boers et al. Making an impact on mortality in rheumatoid arthritis. [See footnote Chapter 3.)

[34] Anders HJ, Vielhauer V. Renal co-morbidity in patients with rheumatic diseases. Arthrit Res Ther. 2011 Jun 29 [cited 2017 Mar 18];13:222. Available from: http://arthritis-research.com/content/pdf/ar3256.pdf

[35] Hickson LJ, Crowson CS, Gabriel SE, McCarthy JT, Matteson EL. Development of reduced kidney function in rheumatoid arthritis. Am J Kidney Dis. 2014 Feb [cited 2017 Mar 18]63(2):206-213. Available from: https://www.ncbi.nlm.nih.gov/pmc/articles/pmid/24100126/

[36] Abedin S. 10 serious RA symptoms. (See footnote in Chapter 1.)

[37] Wilke WS. Rheumatoid arthritis. (See footnote Chapter 5.)

[38] Zoto A. Ocular involvement in patients with rheumatoid arthritis. (See footnote Chapter 4.)

[39] Artifoni M, Rothschild PR, Brézin A, Guillevin L, Puéchal X. Ocular inflammatory diseases associated with rheumatoid arthritis. Nat Rev Rheumatol. 2014 Feb [cited 2017 Jul 11];10(2):108-16. DOI: 10.1038/nrrheum.2013.185

[40] Michaud K, Wolfe F. Comorbidities in rheumatoid arthritis. Best Pract Res Cl Rh. 2007 Oct 21 [cited 2017 May 5];21(5):885-906. DOI: 10.1016/j.berh.2007.06.002

[41] Mayo Clinic [website]. Swollen lymph nodes. 2016 Oct 26 [cited 2017 Jul 15]. Available from: http://www.mayoclinic.org/diseases-conditions/swollen-lymph-nodes/symptoms-causes/dxc-20258981

[42] Medline Plus, National Library of Medicine [website]. Swollen lymph nodes. 2016 Jan 10 [cited 2017 Jul 2]. Available from: https://medlineplus.gov/ency/article/003097.htm

[43] Motulsky AG, Weinberg S, Saphir O, Rosenberg E. Lymph nodes in rheumatoid arthritis. AMA Arch Intern Med. 1952 [cited 2017 Jul 15];90(5):660–676. DOI:10.1001/archinte.1952.00240110086009

[44] M Çalgüneri, MA Öztürk, Z Özbalkan, A Akdogan, K Üreten, S Kiraz, I Ertenli. Frequency of lymphadenopathy in rheumatoid arthritis and systemic lupus erythematosus. J Int Med Res. 2003 Aug 1 [cited 2017 Jul 17] 31(4): 345-349. DOI: 10.1177/147323000303100415

[45] Aktekin LA, Gözlükaya H, Bodur H, Borman P, Köz O. Peripheral neuropathy in rheumatoid arthritis patients: An electroneurophysiological study. Turk J Rheumatol. 2009 [cited 2017 Jul 22];24(2);062-066. Available from: http://

www.archivesofrheumatology.org/full-text-pdf/293

[46] Oláh C, Kardos Z, Sepsi M, Sas A, Kostyál L, Bhattoa HP, Hodosi K, Kerekes G, Tamási L, Valikovics A, Bereczki D, Szekanecz Z. Assessment of intracranial vessels in association with carotid atherosclerosis and brain vascular lesions in rheumatoid arthritis. Arthrit Res Ther. 2017 Sep 26 [cited 2017 Sep 26];19:213. Available from: https://doi.org/10.1186/s13075-017-1422-x

[47] Kardos Z, Oláh C, Sepsi M, Sas A, Kostyál L, Bóta T, Bhattoa H, Hodosi K, Kerekes G, Tamási L, Bereczki D, Szekanecz Z, unpublished data, 2017 Sep [cited 2017 Sep 26].

[48] Newman T. Liver function: What does the liver do? Medical News Today [website], 2016 Feb 15 [cited 2017 Jul 22]. Available from: http://www.medicalnewstoday.com/articles/305075.php

[49] Yunt ZX. Lung disease in rheumatoid arthritis. (See footnote Chapter 2.)

[50] Fleming A, Dodman S, et al. Extra-articular features in early rheumatoid disease. (See footnote in Chapter 1.)

[51] Abraham S, Begum S, Isenberg D. Hepatic manifestations of autoimmune rheumatic diseases. Ann Rheum Dis. 2004 [cited 2017 Jul 22];63:123–129. DOI: 10.1136/ard.2002.001826

[52] Selmi C, De Santis M, Gershwin ME. Liver involvement in subjects with rheumatic disease. Arthritis Res Ther. 2011 Jun 30 [cited 2017 Jul 20];(13):226. Available from: https://doi.org/10.1186/ar3319

[53] Selmi et al. Liver involvement. (See footnote Chapter 6.)

[54] Cojocaru M, Cojocaru IM, Silosi I, Vrabie CD. Liver involvement in patients with systemic autoimmune diseases. Mædica. 2013 Oct 22 [cited 2017 Jul 22];8(4):394-397. Available from: https://www.ncbi.nlm.nih.gov/pmc/articles/PMC3968480/

[55] Cojocaru et al. Liver involvement in patients with systemic. (See footnote Chapter 6.)

[56] Dhikav V, Singh S, Pande S, Chawla A, Anand KS. Non-steroidal drug-induced gastrointestinal toxicity: Mechanisms and management. JIACM 2003 [cited 2017 Jul 22];4(4):315-22. Available from: http://medind.nic.in/jac/t03/i4/jact03i4p315.pdf

[57] Boers et al. Making an impact on mortality in rheumatoid arthritis. (See footnote Chapter 3.)

[58] Myasoedova E, Matteson EL, Talley NJ, Crowson CS. Increased incidence and impact of upper and lower gastrointestinal events in patients with rheumatoid arthritis in Olmsted County, Minnesota: A longitudinal population-based study. J Rheumatol. 2012 July [cited 2017 Jul 22];39(7):1355-1362. Available from: https://www.ncbi.nlm.nih.gov/pmc/articles/PMC3389143/

[59] Harvard Health Publications [website]. Harvard Medical School. Arthritis associated with inflammatory bowel disease. 2014 Oct [cited 2017 Jul 25]. Available from: https://www.health.harvard.edu/digestive-health/arthritis-associated-with-inflammatory-bowel-disease

[60] Haridas V, Malladad G, Haridas K. Co-occurrence of rheumatoid arthritis with ulcerative colitis: A rare case. IJRCI. 2016 Mar 18 [cited 2017 Jul 25]4(1):CS1. Available from: https://www.chanrejournals.com/index.php/rheumatology/article/view/173/html

[61] NYU Langone Medical Center, New York University School of Medicine. Intestinal bacteria linked to rheumatoid arthritis. Science Daily [website]. 2013 Nov 5 [cited 2017 Jul 15]. Available from: https://www.sciencedaily.com/releases/2013/11/131105132031.htm

[62] Scher JU, Sczesnak A, Longman RS, Segata N, Ubeda C, Bielski C, Rostron T, Cerundolo V, Pamer EG, Abramson SB, et al. Expansion

of intestinal Prevotella copri correlates with enhanced susceptibility to arthritis. Author response 9. eLife Sciences, Human Biology and Medicine. 2013 Nov 5 [cited 2017 Jul 26]2:e01202. Available from: https://elifesciences.org/articles/01202#sthash.b3jK5FW4.dpuf

[63] NYU Langone Medical Center. Intestinal bacteria linked to rheumatoid arthritis. (See footnote Chapter 6.)

[64] National Institute of Arthritis and Musculoskeletal and Skin Diseases [website]. Handout on health: Rheumatoid arthritis. 2009 Apr 15 [cited 2013 Apr 28]. Available from: http://www.niams.nih.gov/Health_Info/Rheumatic_Disease/

[65] Cleveland Clinic [website]. Rheumatoid arthritis. 2009 Aug 3 [cited 2013 Apr 28]. Available from: http://my.clevelandclinic.org/orthopaedics-rheumatology/diseases-conditions/hic-rheumatoid-arthritis.aspx

[66] Centers for Disease Control and Prevention. Rheumatoid arthritis. (See footnote Chapter 3.)

[67] WebMD [website]. Rheumatoid arthritis overview. 2012 Apr 30 [cited 2013 Apr 28]. Available from: http://www.webmd.com/rheumatoid-arthritis/guide/rheumatoid-arthritis-basics

[68] Arthritis Foundation. Rheumatoid arthritis fact sheet. (See footnote Chapter 2.)

[69] Simon H. Rheumatoid arthritis – Symptoms. University of Maryland Medical Center [website]. 2009 Feb 19 [cited 2013 Apr 28]. Available from http://www.umm.edu/patiented/articles/what_symptoms_of_rheumatoid_arthritis_000048_4.htm

[70] Matsen F, Leopold SS, Gardner GC, editors. Rheumatoid arthritis. University of Washington Orthopedics and Sports Medicine [website] 2001 Feb 1 [cited 2013 Apr 29]. Available from: http://www.orthop.washington.edu/?q=patient-care/articles/arthritis/

rheumatoid-arthritis.html

[71] Tidy C. Rheumatoid arthritis. Patient.co.uk [website]. 2012 Feb 21 [cited 2013 May 5]. Available from: http://www.patient.co.uk/health/rheumatoid-arthritis

[72] Dooren JC. FDA panel recommends approval of Pfizer's tofacitinib. (See footnote Chapter 2.)

[73] Dooren JC. FDA approves rheumatoid arthritis drug. 2010 Jan 8 [cited 2016 Mar 4]. Available from: http://www.wsj.com/articles/SB10001424052748703481004574647043269341458

[74] Dooren JC. FDA panel recommends approval of Pfizer's tofacitinib. Euroinvestor. 2012 Sep 5 15:30 ET [cited 2013 Apr 28]. Available from: www.euroinvestor.fr/actualites/2012/05/09/fda-panel-recommends-approval-of-pfizerampaposs-tofacitinib/11987854

[75] Seetharaman M. Rheumatoid arthritis: In and out of the joint. (See footnote Chapter 2.)

[76] Eustice C. Rheumatoid arthritis or rheumatoid disease — Does the name really matter? What matters and what doesn't. About.com [website] 2016 Feb 2 [cited 2016 Mar 4]. Available from: http://arthritis.about.com/od/rheumatoidarthritis/fl/Rheumatoid-Arthritis-or-Rheumatoid-Disease-Does-the-Name-Really-Matter.htm

[77] Pincus T, Callahan L. Taking mortality in rheumatoid arthritis seriously – Predictive markers, socioeconomic status and comorbidity. J Rheumatol. 1986 [cited 2017 Mar 11];13:841-5

[78] Kaplan D. The age of death of parents of patients with rheumatoid arthritis. J Rheumatol. 1986 [cited 2017 Mar 11];13:903-906

[79] Wolfe F, Mitchell DM, Sibley JT, Fries JF, Bloch DA, Williams CA, Spitz PW, Haga M, Kleinheksel SM, Cathey MA. The mortality of

rheumatoid arthritis [abstract]. Arthritis Rheum. 1994 Apr [cited 2013 Apr 29];37(4):481-94. Available from: http://www.ncbi.nlm.nih.gov/pubmed/8147925

[80] Fleming A, Dodman S, et al. Extra-articular features in early rheumatoid disease. (See footnote in Chapter 1.)

[81] Kuller LH, Mackey RH, Walitt BT, Deane KD, Holers VM, Robinson WH, Sokolove J, Chang Y, Liu S, Parks CG, et al. Determinants of mortality among postmenopausal women in the Women's Health Initiative who report rheumatoid arthritis. Arthritis Rheum. 2014 Apr 28[cited 2017 Mar 5];66(5):497–507. DOI: 10.1002/art.38268

[82] Listing et al. Mortality in rheumatoid arthritis. (See footnote Chapter 3.)

[83] Jones C. Death by rheumatoid arthritis. (See footnote Chapter 2.)

[84] McLeod M. Deborah Norville in the dynamic Deborah Norville. Modern Senior Living Magazine. 2009 Jan 7 [cited 2012 Apr 14].

[85] PR Newswire [website]. New York. Deborah Norville launches National Hope Relay in celebration of people leading active lives despite their rheumatoid arthritis. 2003 May 28 [cited 2016 Mar 4]. Available from: http://www.prnewswire.com/news-releases/deborah-norville-launches-national-hope-relay-in-celebration-of-people-leading-active-lives-despite-their-rheumatoid-arthritis-71134462.html

[86] Fox M. Adrienne Rich, influential feminist poet, dies at 82. New York Times [Internet]. 2012 Mar 28 [cited 2013 Apr 14]. Available from: http://www.nytimes.com/2012/03/29/books/adrienne-rich-feminist-poet-and-author-dies-at-82.html

[87] Young K. Glenn Frey's cause of death. Rheumatoid Arthritis Warrior [website]. 2016 Jan 20 [cited 2016 Dec 10]. Available from:

http://rawarrior.com/glenn-freys-cause-of-death/

[88] Lynch L. Eagles manager says Glenn Frey's death caused partly by medications. Billboard [website]. 2016 Jan 19 [cited 2016 Dec 10]. Available from: http://www.billboard.com/articles/news/6844175/glenn-frey-death-eagles-medication-irving-azoff

[89] Kimura Y, Weiss JE, Haroldson KL, Lee T, Punaro M, Oliveira S, Rabinovich E, Riebschleger M, Antón J, Blier PR, et al. Pulmonary hypertension and other potentially fatal pulmonary complications in systemic juvenile idiopathic arthritis. Arthrit Care Res. 2013 Apr 3 [cited 2017 Mar 14]. Available from: http://onlinelibrary.wiley.com/doi/10.1002/acr.21889/full

CHAPTER SEVEN
A DOCTOR ADDRESSES THE RA IDENTITY CRISIS

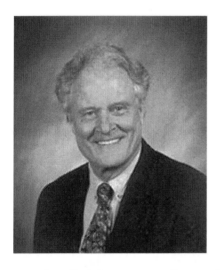

Dr. Frank Adams sounds much like patients when discussing the vocabulary of RA. He wrote the article "An Identity Crisis for RA" in 2011, sharing experiences as a practicing community rheumatologist. The combination of his poetic tone and passionate voice captivated me as a patient-journalist. As you will see below, Dr. Adams is eager to see change and supportive of patient efforts to update the name of RA.

Dr. Adams is clinical associate professor of medicine at the University of Tennessee Health Science Center and a clinical rheumatologist at The Arthritis Group, P.C. in Memphis. Deep appreciation is acknowledged to Dr. Adams for permission to reprint his article. I am grateful to Dr. Adams for granting permission to reprint his article.

An Identity Crisis for RA:

A few suggestions to bring rheumatic disease the recognition and respect it deserves

The following article was originally printed in The Rheumatologist.[1]

by R. Franklin Adams, MD

Despite the numerous advances in treating rheumatic diseases over the past few decades, a major communication gap still exists in the community regarding the complexity and gravity of rheumatic diseases. The reality is that, in spite of the well-intended efforts of the ACR and the Arthritis Foundation (AF), the average lay individual still has only a limited concept of what systemic, inflammatory arthritis is all about.

Who among our citizenry believes that, on any given day in the future, he or she could suddenly wake up with a dozen or so hot, swollen joints radiating intense pain throughout the body, an inflammation which might literally continue for the rest of the individual's life? Most healthy persons don't realize such dramatic events even happen, much less that they have a conceivable risk for it happening to them. Instead, the wrong messages continue to permeate the public's psyche. Virtually any day of the week, you find some reference in the media to "Avoid arthritis, take vitamins, and exercise!" How offended our patients with rheumatoid arthritis (RA) must feel when they see this deceptive advertising. It's inconceivable that patients in this day and age should be made to feel shame or guilt for "having allowed" this devastating disease to happen to their bodies! In the popular culture of the day, RA hardly merits disease status, and is very often cast commonly as a stress-induced "condition" or a vitamin deficiency.

RA is so typically out of the mainstream consciousness that, whenever healthy persons do develop an acute inflammatory disease, their instincts lead them to believe that whatever is happening to them is far removed from "arthritis." And typically, when given a diagnosis of rheumatoid arthritis, patients tend to be nonplussed and sometimes even irate. "No, you must not understand what I'm telling you. This isn't rheumatism, I am in excruciating pain!" And so it goes—many times over.

Lack of Public Knowledge

Unless we plan on curing these terrible illnesses in the near future, I suggest we take a serious look at how to best inform the public and the entire healthcare establishment of the incredible seriousness of rheumatic diseases, and get as far away as possible from a trivial concept of "arthritis." Our patients should receive the best possible care and treatment from us, certainly, but they also want and deserve, as Aretha Franklin said, "R-E-S-P-E-C-T" from their family, friends, and peers. It is we professionals, not the patients, who should be making clear to the public the severe, catastrophic nature of diseases such as RA and the toll they take on society.

To the extent we have not adequately done so, we have not been fair stewards to the very patients that we have dedicated our lives to serving. We should do a better public-relations (PR) job on our patients' behalf, and also on our profession's behalf. Indeed, the better the job of PR we do for our patients, the more prominent our standing as a profession becomes in society—a win-win proposition.

Language Lacks Impact

Standard rheumatology terms such as "inflammatory," "erosive," or even "rheumatoid," add very little special meaning or understanding to the average patient's concept of arthritis. People tend to associate "inflammatory" with infection, and "erosive" more commonly with corrosive, as in wear-and-tear arthritis. And while it is a major medical decision for the rheumatologist to classify a patient as "rheumatoid," to many patients, the term still sounds like "rheumatism" and not what they want—or expect—to hear.

Indeed, after explaining to a recent patient that he did have RA, I was chagrined when he looked up and said, "I've never heard of any arthritis hurting this bad, and now you are telling me it's incurable. Are you guys trying to keep this stuff a secret, or something?"

Newly diagnosed RA patients don't want to have a catastrophic diagnosis like cancer, but they do expect whatever is causing their problem to at least garner some measure of understanding and respect from their family and peers. They want to hear an explanation for their suffering that is accountable not just for their misery, but also for their inability to function and to take care of their families and their careers. Their a priori concept of "arthritis" doesn't fit this bill. To the uninitiated, the term "arthritis," with or without the "rheumatoid" prefix, seems inadequate and understates their problem.

At the other end of the patient spectrum is the chronic, lifelong, RA patient. I am continually impressed with the fortitude that typical longstanding rheumatoid patients display, year after year. It's incredible how tolerant and steadfast they become in dealing with their pain and misery. Perhaps they've reached the point where they feel that their complaints fall on deaf ears, and this is their dignified manner of dealing with a strange curse that nobody on the outside understands or appreciates.

Thus, both RA groups are frustrated: the new-onset, acute patient is incredulous that such a terrible disease goes unappreciated and unrecognized, and the chronic patients have withdrawn into a shell and a long, endless survival mode. Aside from all the pain, RA can also prove to be quite lonely.

In sum, I believe that we have not adequately prepared the public for the potential calamity of developing RA. Regrettably, the disease has very little identity unto its own. Despite all the good efforts and intentions of the ACR and the AF, the average individual still has very little appreciation for the vast differences between the two polar opposites: osteoarthritis (OA) and RA. There is no sense of proportionality between the two, no perspective. Only those stricken with the latter quickly learn to distinguish it from the former, the hard way.

Nomenclature

Confusion of nomenclature remains, in large part, for this failure of insight. Surely, at some point, we should admit mission: impossible! The current classification is simply too archaic and uninformative to expect nonprofessionals to comprehend. Its one thing to teach medical students to distinguish between OA and RA, but its quite another to expect the media or the public to "get it." It's past time that we should consider making changes for the sake of clarity for both our patients and the public.

Verbiage and nomenclature certainly do matter. Recently, one of my more erudite golfing buddies asked me (with only a bit of tongue in cheek), "What is it you rheuma-tologists study, phlegm?"

We must face the reality that anything with "arthritis" as part of its name is likely to be relegated to a second tier of human suffering. And, as aforementioned, adding the prefix "rheumatoid" frequently adds little additional impact or insight. Looking back, I believe humanity would have been better served had our forefathers originally designated RA as "rheumatic arthritis" rather than "rheumatoid" (i.e., rheumatic-like) to distinguish it from rheumatic fever. The "rheumatic" connotation would imply a more dynamic and potentially serious illness and would have better distinguished it from OA. "Rheumatoid" sounds indolent, retiring, and yes, more like "rheumatism."

A Humble Suggestion

As an initial salvo towards better understanding for all, I suggest it is time for some simple, but significant, name changes. The current nomenclature is simply too arcane and misleading. We are using 18th century nomenclature for 21st century bioscience. We are dealing with catastrophic disease here, under the guise of "rheumatism." It just doesn't make good sense, and I feel is no longer appropriate.

It's probably too much to ask to officially change the RA title outright, but I do hereby humbly recommend that we make a small step toward clarification by officially adding the descriptive prefix of autoimmune to the RA label: ARA. "Autoimmune" is one of the few reasonably *avant garde* terms that has caught some viable traction in the media. An additional option would be to faze RA into the more compelling rheumatic arthritis, (which has a precedent vis-à-vis psoriatic arthritis), or even a combination of the two descriptive nouns.

These type of name changes—and I'm sure there are other possibilities—could help give distinction and substance to the disease, and give due justice to those who have suffered too long with too little empathy and insight under the bland "rheumatoid" label. **The important goal is to make it quite clear to the public that we are not dealing with a condition here, but a disease, a rheumatic disease, and a very serious one at that.**

Empower The Public!

Whatever the nomenclature, I truly get the feeling that the general public is anxious to learn more properly what autoimmune inflammatory diseases are about, and we need not disappoint them. Specifically, the public deserves basic knowledge to understand how rheumatic diseases are inflammatory, but not infectious, and that most types have been proven to be driven by an out-of-control immune system —not "too low" immunity, but an over active, autoimmune state. Also, we should be sharing and teaching some of our key operative phrases, such as systemic inflammatory, anti-inflammatory, immune mediated, drug-induced, etc. with the public as well.

Patients surely deserve to be better informed about the basic process of their disease. We can't have patients feeling guilt or shame for their misery and their inability to function in society. To avoid this, we need to better endow them with the basic knowledge of what is happening to their bodies, and to give them the verbal tools to be able to share this information with others. And, surely, to educate them and their families that they didn't do anything "wrong" to deserve their fate.

Ultimately, these same messages are what we need to get through to the public as well. To wit, it's a rare occasion when one encounters a treatise that genuinely attempts to explain to the public the intricate and serious nature of autoimmune and/or inflammatory arthritis and how, once unleashed, an autoimmune rheumatic process can lead to an unrelenting downhill course of pain and autodestruction of joints and body tissues. Consequently, if the public and the powers that be (including third-party insurers) don't have respect for the complexity and gravity of a disease, how could they possibly have respect for the profession treating that disease? And, yes, to cut to the quick, reimbursement for treating such unheralded disease is not likely to lead the pack.

Following this same construct, I feel it was a tactical error years ago when many rheumatology charities were lumped under the heading of the Arthritis Foundation (AF). I truly believe the AF has done a remarkable job, especially working under the generic label of "arthritis." In retrospect, society might have been better served had "rheumatic disease" been the headline cause, as opposed to "arthritis" alone. This would be analogous to the field of neurology specifying individual foundations for its epilepsy, multiple sclerosis, and muscular dystrophy drives as opposed to a single "neuro" foundation.

It's not that I don't have sympathy for all types of arthritis, but I believe the singular "arthritis" title conjures images other than that which we are supporting. I suspect it might be easier to arouse more support for a foundation that also included rheumatic disease, and perhaps end up with more funds to distribute among all of the various types of arthritis. And, importantly, we would be putting the "rheumatic" name front and center in the nation's conscience.

I hereby propose that we suggest to our dedicated and peripatetic sister organization, the Arthritis Foundation, that it consider extending its official title more specifically to include systemic diseases, hence to become the Arthritis and Rheumatic Disease Foundation. I know I am treading on hallowed ground here, but in the long run, I feel this name enhancement would prove extremely beneficial to this great foundation.

Embrace Rheumatology

On a final personal note, I would like to add that becoming a rheumatologist was the best career decision I ever made, and I'm extremely proud of the accomplishments of our specialty. Rheumatology is one of the most challenging and sophisticated of all subspecialties of medicine, and is in large part responsible for having unraveled the extreme complexities of the body's immune system and, in turn, autoimmune rheumatic diseases. We need to share both this complexity and the seriousness of autoimmune disease with society in general and attack the ignorance head on. We owe the public more clarity and respect. There is a thin line between fear mongering and informative counseling and, as a professional society, I feel we have erred too cautiously.

We need to stand up, embrace our profession, and explain its mission better to the public: Namely, that as rheumatologists we do treat "arthritis," but it's not our *raison d'être*. We are here to treat systemic rheumatic diseases, and the world needs to know it!

Lastly, in the twilight of a 40-year career as a clinical rheumatologist, "studying phlegm," I do hereby declare myself, with all due respect to my peers and associates, not an I.D. or Infectious Disease specialist, but an R.D.—a Rheumatic Disease specialist—for now and forevermore.

COMMENTARY

What to do when "RA hardly merits disease status"

When I first read Dr. Adams' piece, I was truly astounded. It's not very often that I read a magazine article and then pick up a phone to track down the author. But I did. And I was similarly surprised by the response of Dr. Adams to me. He was thrilled to receive news of the newly formed RPF, and we have kept in touch over the past couple of years. He encouraged me to write a letter to the editor of The Rheumatologist in response to his article (reproduced at the end of this chapter).

Dr. Adams is precisely correct when he says "rheumatoid" is the "prefix" to "arthritis," which is "inadequate and understates their problem." This phrase could possibly summarize this entire book. As my friend Dave deBronkart said, in this grammatical structure, "rheumatoid" is the adjective, and "arthritis" is the noun.[2] *So, what this expression tells people is "This entity is just a type of arthritis;" "Swollen joints are what it's about;" "What you see is what you get."*

One of the great obstacles faced by PRD is the fact that others usually fail to grasp the reality of the disease—or even that there is a disease. The callousness with which PRD are often treated is a problem that most, except those with the mildest form of the disease, have encountered. Dr. Adams' words are full of compassion for people who are regularly blamed for their illness: "It's inconceivable that patients in this day and age should be made to feel shame or guilt for 'having allowed' this devastating disease to happen to their bodies! In the popular culture of the day, RA hardly merits disease status, and is very often cast commonly as a stress-induced 'condition' or a vitamin deficiency."

I have not argued in this book or elsewhere for a name change solely on that basis, the basis of compassion.

However, it is worth a moment to contemplate how replacing the faulty "arthritis" label could aid and arouse consideration and respect for PRD. Many patients say they disdain the public's reaction to their illness; it is one of the awful problems they face. Whether they are chastised for using handicapped parking spaces or offered vitamin cures at every family function, they find little consolation except among fellow sufferers. Managing a multi-faceted painful chronic disease is certainly made more difficult by others' inappropriate and insensitive responses.

My argument for a name change does not rest on the basis of compassion, although it is merited. Instead, I have argued that there is a great harm that grows from the misnomer: the lack of adequate response from those with the authority to dispense medical care or other necessary support. Dr. Adams hints at the problem near the end of his article when he alludes to money. It's helpful to acknowledge the obvious fact that "the public," whom Adams rightly says must be educated, includes everyone —not just unsympathetic friends and family.

Consider how the fate of PRD is affected by public opinion of the disease:

- The public includes insurance personnel who categorize PRD requests differently than similar requests for comparable diseases.

- The public includes public officials who write policies making it more difficult for PRD to receive needed medications, or even participate in charitable programs offered by the pharmaceutical industry.

- The public includes employers who will not make

appropriate accommodations so that PRD can continue to work as long as possible.

- The public includes judges who routinely deny disability requests for PRD.

- The public includes government officials who consistently underfund research or advocacy for RD, as compared to disease populations of smaller incidence with comparable mortality rates.[3]

- The public even includes healthcare professionals who were not properly taught about RD.

Money is clearly one problem. People representing well-recognized conditions advocated for the recognition and the accommodations and resources that accompany it. The same must be done for RD, now that they have a voice in the RPF. See Chapter 13 for ways you can help correct the public perception of RD.

Lack of awareness impacts treatment costs

As a patient, I've had several opportunities to educate insurance representatives about RD, and why medications or procedures are needed. When a recommended immunization, biopsy, or lab test is rejected by insurance, I ask whether it would be covered for a more well-known disease population, such as diabetes, lupus, or multiple sclerosis. The answer is often frustrating. One of the three instances in which methotrexate was allowed by insurance in tablet form, but not injectable liquid, led to this exasperating discussion:

Customer service: Can you ask the doctor to prescribe another option?

Me: No, methotrexate is a generic drug; there is not another version.

Customer service: Isn't there an alternative to metrex-re-erer-eate?

Me: No, this is considered the background treatment for the disease. Ninety-five percent of RA patients are prescribed meth-o-trex-ate.

Customer service: Your diagnosis is arthritis? You need injections for arthritis?

Me: No. It's a disease. I have to have these injections as treatment. And they are required to continue with my other treatment as well.

Customer service: But it is arthritis, right?

Me: No. It's not... Look, it doesn't matter. This is just about the cheapest treatment for this disease available. (At that time, the cash price for a ninety-day supply of injectable methotrexate was thirty dollars.) And it's almost universally prescribed. I've taken it for years and you need to cover it.

Customer service: We don't have to cover it because you inject it. We don't cover things you inject at home.

Me: It's always been covered. If it were insulin, would you cover it?

Customer service: But that's a treatment for diabetes. Do you have diabetes?

Me: No, but that's exactly my point. RA is a disease, like diabetes. And methotrexate is the treatment.

Dr. Adams put it so perfectly: "Unless we plan on curing these terrible illnesses in the near future, I suggest we take a serious look at how to best inform the public and the entire healthcare establishment of the incredible seriousness of rheumatic diseases, and get as far away as possible from a trivial concept of 'arthritis.'"

I plan to do all in my power to make a cure nearer in my lifetime. Members of my family have been sadly stricken by some of the conditions described in Chapters 5 and 6. The likelihood that one of my five children will be diagnosed has not escaped me. Two of them have already shown signs.

I would say, and I believe my friend Dr. Frank Adams would agree, that our prospects of accomplishing that cure are greatly increased by getting "as far away as possible from a trivial concept of 'arthritis.'"

Overcoming hurdles created by the "a" word

Even when someone makes an effort to understand, hurdles created by the "a" word are difficult to overcome. One journalist who had a relative with the disease had communicated with me several times, interviewing me twice. Even so, the series of articles he wrote about RD were each published with a typical accompanying image of ninety-year-old wrinkled "arthritic" hands.[4] That is what people (editors, journalists, publishers) think of when they read the word "arthritis." When RD is depicted with imagery of hands, the elderly, or minor aches and pains, the myths are perpetuated. If possible, I hope everyone who reads this book, will set aside preconceptions about "rheumatoid arthritis" and consider the facts presented.

> "WHO AMONG OUR CITIZENRY BELIEVES THAT,
> ON ANY GIVEN DAY IN THE FUTURE, HE OR SHE COULD
> SUDDENLY WAKE UP WITH A DOZEN OR SO HOT, SWOLLEN
> JOINTS RADIATING INTENSE PAIN THROUGHOUT THE BODY,
> AN INFLAMMATION WHICH MIGHT LITERALLY CONTINUE
> FOR THE REST OF THE INDIVIDUAL'S LIFE?"
>
> 2011, R. FRANKLIN ADAMS, M.D.

One question in Dr. Adams' article so accurately portrayed the plight of a PRD, I wondered whether a patient had written it for him: "Who among our citizenry believes that, on any given day in the future, he or she could suddenly wake up with a dozen or so hot, swollen joints radiating intense pain throughout the body, an inflammation which might literally continue for the rest of the individual's life?" In a forty-year career, he must have seen quite a few patients in this predicament. He must have observed patients' shock at how suddenly the disease can disable a person and destroy his or her health.

At times, Adams must have been frustrated at the lack of effective tools available to him to return young patients to health. Perhaps his patients sometimes shared their struggles for understanding or accommodation. Certainly, he was aware of discrepancies in medical coverage for this underserved population. He wrote knowingly: "We need to share both this complexity and the seriousness of autoimmune disease with society in general and attack the ignorance head on. We owe the public more clarity and respect."

The autoimmune dilemma

I agree with Dr. Adams that "Verbiage and nomenclature certainly do matter" and that the current terminology of "arthritis" has done damage to patients and to the profession. In searching for an answer to this problem, Adams recognizes we must be cautious to avoid pitfalls such as the ones he describes that befell the last generation. This same caution guided me as I helped to choose the name for the new RPF late in 2010. After seeking guidance from several advisors, we decided on "Rheumatoid Patient Foundation" which avoided both "a" words, autoimmune and arthritis. Then, in choosing a name to support the effort to make truth more plain to the public, I again considered carefully and sought advice. One expert rheumatologist explained that it is not certain whether all RA is autoimmune in nature since some people do not exhibit antibodies.

It is also likely that what we now know as RA will one day be subdivided into different conditions. We are still very early in the process of comprehending this disease. New research into microbes (see Chapter 1) illustrates the possibility that the theory of autoimmunity could be transformed, at least for some cases.

Patients can sincerely appreciate this desire of a physician to improve the lot of patients with such a harsh disease: "It is we professionals, not the patients, who should be making clear to the public the severe, catastrophic nature of diseases such as RA and the toll they take on society." It is too much for individual patients to take on, but patients are eager for change and enthusiastic to partner with professionals, which we are doing through the RPF.

Since childhood, I've been aware of organizations to advance the cause of diseases such as muscular dystrophy and juvenile diabetes; and in recent years I've learned of numerous organizations for lupus, Sjögren's syndrome, psoriasis, and even or various syndromes with no identified disease process. However until now, as Dr. Adams said, "Regrettably, the disease has very little identity unto its own." The RPF will share that responsibility to educate and to work toward a cure.

The following passage is adapted from an article on rawarrior.com.

RESPONSE TO AN IDENTITY CRISIS FOR RA

Recently, I read an article in *The Rheumatologist* (preceding a new PR campaign by the American College of Rheumatology), "An Identity Crisis for RA: A few suggestions to bring rheumatic disease the recognition and respect it deserves." I strongly recommend that you read the article. It was written by a rheumatologist, but you'll see many points that seem very familiar.

I used *The Rheumatologist's* contact link to send in the following Letter to the Editor. I had contacted Dr. Adams to thank him personally for the article and he suggested I write the Letter to the Editor. Hopefully, they'll publish my letter.

Dear Editors at *The Rheumatologist*:

Thank you for the article "An Identity Crisis for RA; A few suggestions to bring rheumatic disease the recognition and respect it deserves" by R. Franklin Adams, MD (August 2011).

I'd like to quote the article to underscore the parts I liked best, but I'd quote almost the entire piece. If only the whole article could be condensed onto a t-shirt! (See image below.)

Over the last three years, I've written about 800 articles about RA, published on my website and other venues. I've read hundreds of news stories, academic articles, and patient blogs. Meanwhile, I've received at least 200,000 responses directly from RA patients while living full-time with the disease myself.

What have I discovered?

Being lumped with "arthritis," RA has no identity. Patients have already dropped the "a" word and begun to refer to RA as rheumatoid disease. Statistics for mortality rates and research funding are terrible. The problem is as Adams clearly sees it and profoundly states it:

"Who among our citizenry believes that, on any given day in the future, he or she could suddenly wake up with a dozen or so hot, swollen joints radiating intense pain throughout the body, an inflammation which might literally continue for the rest of the individual's life?...Virtually any day of the week, you find some reference in the media to 'Avoid arthritis, take vitamins, and exercise!' How offended our patients with rheumatoid arthritis (RA) must feel when they see this deceptive advertising. It's inconceivable that patients in this day and age should be made to feel shame or guilt for 'having allowed' this devastating disease to happen to their bodies!"

I had made very similar statements to ACR Rheumatology Research Foundation's Steve Echard at the last American College of Rheumatology annual scientific meeting in Atlanta. As I read Dr. Adams' article, I heard my own words echoed. It seemed like he had read the articles that I have written about RA, even a very old one on *Healthcare Professionals Live*.[5] In reality, Dr. Adams and I had no contact before I called him last week.

Astonishingly, by way of different roads, we have come to the same conclusions: RA is a serious disease that is misunderstood by most people, including many professional people and medical personnel. According to Mayo Clinic research, the lifetime risk of developing RA is 3.6% for women and 1.7% for men. For the sake of RA patients and everyone in society (potential RA patients and their loved ones), change must come now.

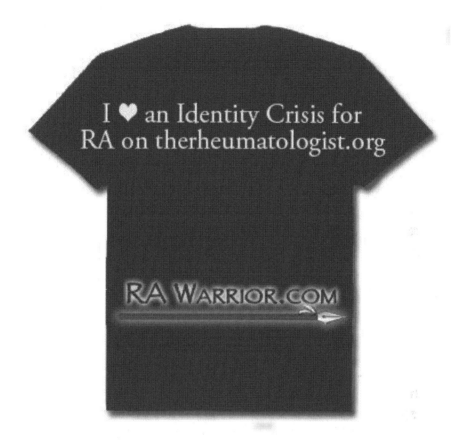

Adams mentions key strategies that have also been advocated by patients through the RA Warrior community, especially RA nomenclature issues. I believe the most successful approach will be one that allows patients, researchers, and doctors to combine efforts to attack the problem of RA on every level (both its identity and its cure).

The first non-profit organization for RA, the Rheumatoid Patient Foundation (RPF), founded in 2011, is dedicated to this purpose. With greater public awareness will come appropriate recognition, research funding, and programs to improve the lives of people with RA.

If there is anything that could be more encouraging to me as a friend and advocate of RA patients than to read this article written by a rheumatologist, it is the response of Dr. Adams to the RPF. He indicated that the work of the RPF is welcome and long overdue in the "rheumatology nation."

Will you also stand with us through rheum4us.org? Everyone interested in improving the lives of RA patients is welcome to become a member. I hope that many physicians will lend support so that together we can create the groundswell of change that will help us to defeat the monster that we call RA.

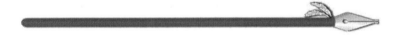

KEY POINTS

1. Dr. Adams: Most people have no idea that they could suddenly be struck with a disease radiating intense pain for the rest of their lives.

2. Dr. Adams: Patients should not be blamed for "having allowed" this devastating disease to happen to their bodies.

3. Dr. Adams: Due to the incredible seriousness of the disease, we must get far away from the trivial concept of "arthritis."

4. Dr. Adams: It doesn't make sense to have a catastrophic disease under the guise of "rheumatism."

5. Rheumatology lacks rightful prestige and finances due to misperceptions of rheumatic disease.

Action step: Rheumatology must throw off misperceptions

and old labels for RD and embrace a more modern and accurate model of RD.

Quote to remember: "The important goal is to make it quite clear to the public that we are not dealing with a condition here, but a disease, a rheumatic disease, and a very serious one at that."

---

[1] Adams RF. An identity crisis for RA. (See footnote Introduction.)

[2] deBronkart D. In Will Venus Williams' Sjögren's syndrome. (See footnote in Chapter 1.)

[3] American College of Rheumatology. Atlanta, GA. Rheumatoid arthritis impacts millions of Americans but remains severely underfunded (consumer media press release). 2007 Jul 12 [cited 2013 Jun 22]. Available from: http://www.prnewswire.com/news-releases/rheumatoid-arthritis-impacts-millions-of-americans-but-remains-severely-underfunded-52732482.html

[4] Martinez J. What exactly is rheumatoid arthritis? Not many know, says one patient. Southern California Public Radio [website]. 2013 Jan 22 [cited 2016 Mar 4]. Available from: http://www.oncentral.org/news/2013/01/22/what-exactly-is-rheumatoid-arthritis-not-many-know/

[5] Young K. Early treatment of rheumatoid arthritis is an elusive goal. Healthcare Professionals Live [website]. 2009 [cited 2012 Oct 1]. Available from: http://www.hcplive.com/articles/early_treatment_of_RA

CHAPTER EIGHT
BENEFITS TO RHEUMATOLOGY

Acknowledging the dangers of rheumatoid disease informs the world in ways that significantly benefit rheumatology.

Limiting RD to "a type of arthritis" impairs rheumatology

The medical field, particularly rheumatology, will benefit considerably from a well-defined model of rheumatoid disease as opposed to rheumatoid arthritis or rheumatism. Many who work in rheumatology clinics or investigation have responded positively to the idea of an official shift toward "rheumatoid disease." It's understandable that rheumatologists become uncomfortable referring to the complex systemic disease as "arthritis," so it is common for rheumatologists to substitute "the rheumatoid," "the disease," or "RA disease" when speaking to patients or in scientific writing. Even fifty years ago, in his classic plea for the recognition of distal interphalangeal (DIP) joints in RA, McCarty only used "rheumatoid arthritis" when referring specifically to joints, and "rheumatoid disease" when referring to the disease generally.[1]

Some specific aspects of the profession that will be positively impacted by a shift in focus and terminology include addressing the rheumatology workforce shortage,[2] insufficient numbers of new doctors entering the profession, insufficient research dollars, academic misperceptions, and inadequate regard from the public. With great flair, Dr. Adams expressed a summary of the current predicament of rheumatology: "It's past time that we should consider making changes for the sake of clarity for both our patients and the public. Verbiage and nomenclature certainly do matter. Recently, one of my more erudite golfing buddies asked me (with only a bit of tongue in cheek), 'What is it you rheuma-tologists study, phlegm?'"

Communication will improve

Communication is certainly a key to medical intervention and treatment. And vocabulary is central to communication between patients and doctors, medical students and professors, as well as consumers and agencies that administrate healthcare dollars. Let's look at how the simple change of dropping the word *arthritis* could have far-reaching effects.

John M. Davis, Mayo Clinic professor and practicing rheumatologist, believes improving communication by changing the name of rheumatoid arthritis will positively impact patients and professionals. "There is a need to change the name of RA. I've learned from patients and others to have a growing appreciation that the words 'rheumatoid arthritis' do not do justice to this disease." He explains that a name that is more reflective of the systemic nature and the mechanisms of the disease ought to be used. According to Davis, all parties in medical care can benefit directly from the name change because "It will help doctors and patients to be able to communicate better. It will also be easier for me to teach about the disease to medical students if there is a name that lives up to the full aspects of the disease." He also believes that updating the name of RA will improve awareness of the nature of the disease: "We will be able to enhance awareness of the disease, what it is, and what it means to people."

Third-party payers of healthcare costs often decline procedures or medications for patients whose diagnosis is coded as "arthritis." Patients endure denials or delays as doctors are forced to provide additional evidence for an exception or generate special authorization *for tests or treatments that should be considered routine with RD* such as cardiovascular testing, prescriptions for injectable methotrexate, and recommended vaccinations that precede biologic treatment. Dr. Davis says that it will be better for both patients and physicians when there is no longer a name that is hindered by the false perceptions created by the word *arthritis*: "When we advocate for a treatment to be approved by payers who cover costs, it would be to our advantage if the name reflects what we are dealing with and is not mired in historical misconceptions about the disease."

Cardiovascular testing is a clear example of necessary care that may often be denied. As early as 2005, an article in the *Oxford Journal of Rheumatology* titled "Disease modification and cardiovascular risk reduction: Two sides of the same coin?" stated that "cardiovascular risk reduction should be considered as integral to the control of disease activity in the care plans of patients with RA" since "recent observations indicate that chronic inflammation is not merely associated with accelerated atherosclerosis but that aberrant cellular and humoral immune responses are integral to its pathogenesis."[3] Yet, cardiovascular evaluations for patients with RD that are recommended by experts[4, 5] would typically be deemed unnecessary by most payers, even if physicians knew to authorize them.

It must be clearly communicated that rheumatoid disease is as much a heart disease as a hand disease. As Dr. Adams wrote in

"An Identity Crisis for RA" (see Chapter 7), it is critical that we better inform "the entire healthcare establishment of the incredible seriousness of rheumatic diseases, and get as far away as possible from a trivial concept of 'arthritis.'" What is obviously needed is the straightforward manner of communication that has taken place in the U.S. in recent decades with regard to other diseases or public health concerns such as lupus, diabetes, depression, and tobacco use.

Shortages within rheumatology

Several factors contribute to a mounting shortage in availability of rheumatological care in the U.S., including an aging population, the majority of which will experience age-related degenerative arthritis (also called osteoarthritis or OA). According to a 2007 U.S. Rheumatology Workforce study, the supply of rheumatologists is not increasing with demand due to fixed numbers entering the workforce and to retirements of doctors who are also aging.[6] And according to an updated workforce study published in 2016, the rheumatologist supply was about 1,000 below the level of demand.[7] However, by 2030 supply could exceed demand by over 4,700 as more people seek rheumatology appointments. The gap will be almost twice what it was projected to be in the original study (which predicted that by 2025, the excess demand would be 2,576).

Future demand is difficult to predict. Previous workforce studies have produced inaccurate estimates; however, the recent studies addressed various complexities to improve projections. Furthermore, the rheumatology workforce projections were based on an assumption of equilibrium of supply and demand in 2005. There is consensus among practicing rheumatologists that the shortage is already worrisome, and this is also reflected in the feedback I receive from U.S. patients.

In addition to the expected increase in arthritic conditions due to an aging population, Mayo Clinic has reported an increase in the prevalence of RA,[8] the most common rheumatic disease that is usually treated by rheumatologists, and which strikes people at any age.[9] These trends signal a need for change if people with rheumatoid disease (PRD) are to obtain proper disease treatment and preventive care. It is increasingly important that patients educate themselves about disease management and the various risks associated with their diagnosis and treatments. They must seek appropriate care wherever necessary.

Rheumatology is facing shortages of doctors, nurses, and research dollars. During recent years, there was a recurring shortage of methotrexate,[10] in the U.S., the standard background treatment for RD. There seem to be rheumatology scarcities in everything except patients. The following pages will describe how embracing the term "disease" could positively impact the shortages within rheumatology.

RESEARCH AND ACADEMIC BENEFITS TO RHEUMATOLOGY

Research funding has been low, compared to similar diseases

Lack of awareness about the extent of the disease has resulted in limited research dollars allocated for RA in the U.S. National Institutes of Health (NIH) has historically awarded grants for RA research as a portion of the umbrella category of for arthritis, National Institute of Arthritis and Musculoskeletal and Skin Diseases (NIAMS), while comparable diseases with lower incidence had occupied their own categories. This mislabeling of RD as a type of arthritis impacts granting committees in the same way it influences insurers, media, and the public. As Dr. Adams so clearly explained, "In the popular culture of the day, RA hardly merits disease status." In 2015, RA was added as a category; however, funding remains low in comparison to comparable diseases.

In 2007, the ACR reported research funding allotted for RA is lower than for diseases with similar impact that are more rare: "However, research funding for RA averages as little as $25.90 per patient and remains significantly low compared to other chronic diseases that affect far fewer people like lupus, diabetes and multiple sclerosis, which average $330.00 per patient."[11] This ratio is about .078, approximately one to twelve, or eight percent of the amount spent on similar diseases. In the following years, NIH funding continued this trend in per-patient spending on RA in comparison to SLE, as I calculated in 2012. NIH granted approximately three times as much for lupus as RA, while Mayo Clinic and Hospital for Special Surgery estimate that RD has four or five times the prevalence of lupus, respectively.[12, 13] Again, it was conservatively about a one to twelve ratio of per patient spending, or eight percent as much.

This disparity still exists in 2017, but it is more difficult to quantify. In 2015, NIH created an actual spending category for RA for the first time. An NIH spokesman stated that comparisons cannot be made between current spending and spending before 2015. Current "Research, Condition, and Disease Categorization"on the NIH website appears to reflect a per-patient spending ratio of approximately one to four or one to five for RA and comparable diseases such as SLE and MS.

As Practice Chair of the Division of Rheumatology at Mayo Clinic in Rochester, Minnesota, John Davis believes the connection between poor research funding and disease awareness is clear: "I think the reason funding for rheumatoid disease is historically lower is that (1) it took many years for rheumatology community to become aware and embrace the systemic aspect of the disease in terms of the greater mortality. In recent years, there is a growing awareness of the cardiovascular mortality, malignancies, infections, and changes in body composition related to RA. So that was under-recognized and (2) people think of *arthritis* as not that great of a problem and that it's just something you have to deal with."

"And," Davis adds, "the disease has also been perceived as rarer than it actually is—we have found that in Rochester, Minnesota, the lifetime risk of RA is 3.6% for women and a 1.7% for men. So funding has not risen to the levels of some other chronic diseases. We do need the voice of patients to lobby for awareness." Dr. Davis believes that recognition of the toll on patients' and families' lives, and on communities financially, is one way to get the world's attention. And he is confident that "a name that's more representative of the disease will make it easier to advocate for research funds."

Misperceptions of the disease affect research funding

The misperception that the disease called *rheumatoid arthritis* is merely "a type of arthritis" has had a disturbing effect on investigators' attempts to obtain funds. According to Dr. Rebecca Bader formerly of the Burton Blatt Institute, "The real problem is that people are simply unaware of the seriousness of the disease to begin with, so the funding opportunities in general relative to other things are very limited."

But confusion hinders research for RA at multiple levels. In some instances, RA research is placed into the category of *regenerative medicine* because of what Dr. Bader calls the "arthritis confusion." She says, "People, even well educated people, still believe, regardless of what I say or how I say it, that osteoarthritis and rheumatoid arthritis must be linked since they both contain the word arthritis."

Tissue engineering is a popular translational research topic, but it currently relates more to osteoarthritis because the disease process is localized, rather than rheumatoid, a systemic disease. The goal of this type of research is to learn to replace or even regenerate arthritic tissue. RA cannot effectively compete in this funding environment since current goals of RA research are more basic, such as learning the true etiology of the disease and identifying systemic treatment strategies. "For RA, the money would be far better spent learning more about the disease and how to better target the disease and how to identify individual, effective treatment strategies. Yet, because of the word arthritis, I firmly believe that these particular funding opportunities are not available outside of NIAMS. That is very unfortunate."

And, as noted above, NIH has historically limited rheumatoid disease research funding to an arthritis sub-category within NIAMS. Outside of NIAMS, researchers have actually been discouraged from pursuing funding projects related to rheumatoid disease, as Dr. Bader recalled when interviewed.

Confusion about how to categorize RA academically

Even in elite academic circles, the name of RA leads to misunderstanding. At academic institutions, RA is often grouped with geriatric (aging) research. This confusion about the nature and scope of the disease leads to obstacles in opportunities for research which in turn further limits research funding.

Professor Bader is well aware of this problem. Dr. Bader's lab was dedicated to research on RA for several years. She has a personal connection to the disease, having an aunt who has suffered from it for decades, and therefore she has a more thorough appreciation of it than many do.

Professor Bader has frequently encountered confusion about the nature of RA as a disease. "Because of the dreaded word arthritis, I have been asked on multiple occasions to spin my research such that I can obtain funding opportunities aimed at improving the quality of life of the elderly. Once, after explaining to my colleague that I would not propose something that related to osteoarthritis, a disease that I know relatively little about, nor would I put RA and osteoarthritis together, I was told that I was wrong. Just wrong."

Even after clarifying that RA is not a disease of the elderly, Bader was later asked to research eye problems faced by the elderly and to relate that to RA. Of course, she explained again that the eye issues faced by RA patients are different than eye issues related to the aging process. She describes other experiences with professionals in the scientific research industry where the study of RA is scoffed at as unimportant in relation to cancer or viewed as an insignificant disease. In Dr. Bader's opinion, "Industry does have money that could be directed to RA research, and they are not directing it to the right places because they don't understand how much of a problem it is."

The academic confusion is also evident in the inconsistency of the language used to describe this disease. As dozens of examples in this book demonstrate, "rheumatoid disease" is a historical term that is still used in research literature, especially in publications that primarily address the extra-articular aspects of the disease, such as thoracic journals. However, in an attempt to bridge the gap between today's most common term, "RA" and the reality of a systemic disease, some writers have surprisingly used both terms together, "RA disease."[14, 15, 16, 17, 18] One adjective, rheumatoid, obviously cannot modify two nouns (arthritis and disease); however, such linguistic gymnastics are not unexpected with the confusion that surrounds RD.

Creating an accurate disease identity can increase research opportunities

The prospects for funding will improve as we resolve the crisis of an erroneous understanding of RD and establish a more accurate characterization of it as a disease. First, it could end embarrassing denials of private research dollars that accompany questions of whether RD is an important condition to study, such as encountered by Dr. Bader.

Second, a more accurate public perception of the disease will lead to more balanced public research funding so that spending for RD will be on par with comparable conditions. Of course, increased research dollars will lead to more opportunities for rheumatology investigators, which will attract more people to enter the field.

Finally, creating an accurate awareness of the disease could reduce impediments to research funding that can slow progress toward a cure. As research intensifies, knowledge and awareness of RD will increase further, contributing greater to interest in the field. Interest could reach critical mass and peak the concern for a cure to RD.

ACKNOWLEDGING RHEUMATOID DISEASE TO REVITALIZE RHEUMATOLOGY

Recognition and reimbursement

Nearing the end of a long career in rheumatology, Dr. Frank Adams (see Chapter 7) has witnessed some of the unfolding medical history that is recounted in this book. He clearly recognizes the disconnection between public opinion and the complexity of rheumatic diseases like RD. "Despite the numerous advances in treating rheumatic diseases over the past few decades, a major communication gap still exists in the community regarding the complexity and gravity of rheumatic diseases," he wrote.

Dr. Adams also related the misunderstanding about RD to the lack of recognition and financial inequity in rheumatology: "Consequently, if the public and the powers that be (including third-party insurers) don't have respect for the complexity and gravity of a disease, how could they possibly have respect for the profession treating that disease? And, yes, to cut to the quick, reimbursement for treating such unheralded disease is not likely to lead the pack."

Obviously, a more accurate appraisal of rheumatic inflammatory disease, the most common being RD, could enhance recognition and reimbursement of the professionals who treat it.

Acknowledging the systemic features of RD could also expand the appeal of the profession to prospective doctors. I have heard experienced doctors say a lack of awareness of RD leaves medical students, potential new rheumatologists, with a mistaken impression that rheumatologists only treat the arthritis that is typical of aging. If they *do* have an interest in treating the elderly, they will likely choose gerontology as a field. If they do *not* want to work exclusively with the elderly, young doctors may reject the field rheumatology out of hand, mistakenly believing the field concerns only the aging population. If the confusion surrounding RD cleared, interest in the field would likely rise.

Young men and women with particular interest in treating the elderly will likely already have chosen gerontology as a field, so they may not consider rheumatology either. Interest in rheumatology would unmistakably be cultivated by clearing up the confusion surrounding RD.

Facing the frustration of rheumatology

William Osler, the doctor considered the father of rheumatology, famously said: "When a patient with arthritis comes in the front door, I try to go out the back door."[19] What makes a doctor feel like running from patients? And why did this legendary doctor feel that way about his patients with a difficult disease? There is an undeniable frustration when working in rheumatology.

Many have commented on why, historically, rheumatology has been a discouraging profession: doctors must watch patients with incurable conditions progressively decline. In patients who do not respond well to treatments, joints tend to gradually worsen until they deteriorate enough to require referral to another specialty for surgical repair or replacement. Over the past several years, new drugs have rescued RD from being a hopeless task to a challenging, and sometimes rewarding one. Data from clinical trials constantly show that a minority of PRD have an excellent response to currently available treatments.[20, 21, 22, 23, 24, 25, 26] And, with prevalence of RD estimated at 1 percent (see Chapter 3), millions of people need the help of rheumatologists.

Clinical studies have confirmed what patients know first-hand: clinical or sustained remission is uncommon in RD in ordinary clinic settings.[27, 28, 29, 30, 31] But the emerging approach of *treatment to target* seeks to make remission or low disease activity more attainable, based on the same "tight control" model used successfully in diabetes.[32, 33] Current research priorities include developing new types of treatments to help those who don't respond to currently approved treatments and also discovering ways to identify which treatments will help which patients.

> "MORE EVIDENCE, LESS EMINENCE, ELOQUENCE, AND ELEGANCE WILL ENHANCE RHEUMATOLOGY CARE FOR PATIENTS AND THEIR RHEUMATOLOGISTS."
>
> 2007, PINCUS & TUGWELL

(Footnote.)[34]

Revitalizing rheumatology by making it chic

Dr. Adams said that people sometimes think rheumatologists "study phlegm" and implied that they suffer a resulting lack of respect. It is a colorful way to acknowledge the notion that rheumatology is an irrelevant specialty. Even with his good humor, one can detect his frustration on behalf of his beloved lifelong profession of "rheumatic disease specialist."

While rheumatology may not ever be as profitable as plastic surgery or as highly regarded as neurosurgery, it can certainly be far more esteemed than phlegm! Millions of people have diseases that affect their joints, so rheumatology could become more popular as the public gains better understanding of the variety of conditions these doctors attend to, including complex diseases like RD.

Public relations campaigns attempt to create an attractive image and invite more attention to the profession, highlighting patients who have been helped.[35] This is one approach to addressing the rheumatologist shortage. At least one rheumatologist has called this approach making rheumatology look "sexy."[36] Hopefully, these efforts will attract more interest in the profession.

However, there is only one thing that can make rheumatology truly compelling: success.

In the 1950's, rheumatology was successful, compelling, and chic. Hench and Kendall won a Nobel Prize for the use of cortisone with rheumatoid arthritis. It put Mayo Clinic on the map as people traveled from far and wide to try the new drug. More doctors entered rheumatology. More patients showed up to be treated. RA and the doctors who treated it were out in the open and positively popular for a while.

Unfortunately, lasting and comprehensive success has remained elusive with RA. Early cortisone success developed into a very un-sexy nightmare of "adverse events." When typical clinical trial response rates are presented in a traditional pie chart arrangement, one can see that treatments typically bring 70% improvement to about 20% of patients, bring 50% improvement to about 16% of patients and fail for 34% of patients[37, 38, 39] Overall, about two-thirds of patients have 20% or less improvement. Most improvement is incomplete or temporary as the disease progresses or patients become resistant to medicines.

TYPICAL TREATMENT RESPONSE RATES
(averages from clinical trials)

- 34% no measurable improvement
- 20% get 70% response
- 16% get 50% response
- 29% get 20% response

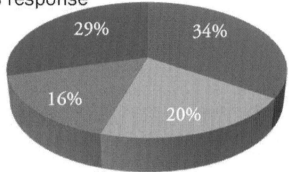

Changing those outcomes will exhilarate rheumatology as it did in the past. Nothing will be more appealing than seeing millions of people desperate for a cure for a devastating disease celebrate because research has succeeded and given them a reprieve from their suffering. Truly, the success of PRD *is* also the success of the doctors who care for them. That success is what makes rheumatology exciting and "sexy."[40]

Dr. John Davis believes doctors recognize that changing the name of RA will benefit them: "I don't think many physicians will argue that the current name is adequate. If we clearly state the need and rationale, it can clearly be done." The need and rationale are apparent: saying "rheumatoid disease" instead of "rheumatoid arthritis" will help both patients and doctors.

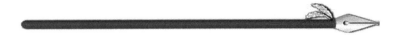

KEY POINTS

1. Rheumatology suffers from inadequate workforce recruits, research funding, financial reimbursement, and public acknowledgment.

2. Dr. Davis: Moving away from the concept of arthritis will help doctors and patients and improve coverage for routine care by enhancing awareness about the disease.

3. Research funding in RD suffers due to misperceptions of RD as a type of arthritis.

4. Public relations campaigns attempt to make rheumatology more attractive, in hope of addressing the shortages.

Action step: Rheumatology should seek success for patients by adopting standards that allow earlier diagnosis and more thorough disease evaluation.

Quote to remember: "However, there is only one thing that can make rheumatology truly compelling: success."

---

[1] McCarty DJ, Gatter RA. A study of distal interphalangeal joint tenderness in rheumatoid arthritis. Arthritis Rheum. 1966 Apr [cited 2013 Aug 21];9(2):325-336. Available from: http://onlinelibrary.wiley.com/doi/10.1002/art.1780090208/pdf

[2] Battafarano D, Monrad S, Fitzgerald J, Bolster M, Deal C, Bass AR, Molina R, Erickson AR, Smith BJ, Jones KB et al. 2015 ACR/ARHP

Workforce study in the United States: Adult rheumatologist supply and demand projections for 2015-2030 [abstract]. Arthritis Rheumatol. 2016 [cited 2017 Mar 24];68(suppl 10). Available from: http://acrabstracts.org/abstract/2015-acrarhp-workforce-study-in-the-united-states-adult-rheumatologist-supply-and-demand-projections-for-2015-2030/

3 Hall FC, Dalbeth N. Disease modification and cardiovascular risk reduction: Two sides of the same coin? (Oxford) Rheumatology. 2005 Dec [cited 2013 Jun 21];44(12):1473-1482. Available from: http://rheumatology.oxfordjournals.org/content/44/12/1473.full

4 Peters MJ, Symmons DP, McCarey D, Dijkmans BA, Nicola P, Kvien TK, McInnes IB, Haentzschel H, Gonzalez-Gay MA, Provan S, et al. EULAR evidence-based recommendations for cardiovascular risk management in patients with rheumatoid arthritis and other forms of inflammatory arthritis. Ann Rheum Dis. 2010 Feb [cited 2013 Feb 20];69(2):325-31. Available from: http://www.ncbi.nlm.nih.gov/pubmed/19773290 DOI: 10.1136/ard.2009.113696

5 Mayo Clinic. Predicting cardiovascular disease risk for rheumatoid arthritis patients. Science Daily [website]. 2007 Nov 11 [cited 2017 Mar 22]. Available from: http://www.sciencedaily.com/releases/2007/11/071107181025.htm

6 Deal CL, Hooker R, Harrington T, Birnbaum N, Hogan P, Bouchery E, Klein-Gitelman M, Barr W. The United States rheumatology workforce: Supply and demand, 2005–2025. Arthritis Rheum. 2007 Mar [cited 2013 Jun 22];56(3):722–729. Available from: http://onlinelibrary.wiley.com/doi/10.1002/art.22437/pdf DOI: 10.1002/art.22437

7 Battafarano et al. 2015 ACR/ARHP Workforce study in the United States. (See footnote Chapter 8.)

8 Myasoedova E, Crowson CS, Kremers HM, Therneau TM, Gabriel

SE. Is the incidence of rheumatoid arthritis rising? Results from Olmsted County, Minnesota, 1955–2007. Arthritis Rheum. 2010 Jun [cited 2031 Jun 22];62(6):1576–1582. Available from: http://onlinelibrary.wiley.com/doi/10.1002/art.27425/full

9 Ruderman E, Tambar S. Rheumatoid arthritis. American College of Rheumatology [website]. 2013 Aug [cited 2016 Mar 4]. Available from: http://www.rheumatology.org/I-Am-A/Patient-Caregiver/Diseases-Conditions/Rheumatoid-Arthritis

10 Young K. Confusion & blame surround methotrexate shortages & recalls. Rheumatoid Arthritis Warrior [website]. 2012 Jul 25 [cited 2013 Mar 23]. Available from: http://rawarrior.com/confusion-and-blame-surround-methotrexate-shortages-recalls/

11 American College of Rheumatology. Rheumatoid arthritis impacts millions. (See footnote Chapter 7.)

12 Mayo clinic determines lifetime risk of adult rheumatoid arthritis. (See footnote Chapter 3.)

13 Hospital for Special Surgery. Hospital for Special Surgery receives grant for new genomics center to study autoimmune diseases (press release). 2013 Apr 25 [cited 2013 May 16]. Available from: http://www.hss.edu/newsroom_genomics-center-study-autoimmune-diseases.asp

14 Iannaccone CK, Lee YC, Cui J, Frits ML, Glass RJ, Plenge RM, Solomon DH, Weinblatt ME, Shadick NA. Using genetic and clinical data to understand response to disease-modifying anti-rheumatic drug therapy: Data from the Brigham and Women's Hospital rheumatoid arthritis sequential study. (Oxford) Rheumatology. 2011 [cited 2017 Mar 22];50(1):40-46. Available from: https://academic.oup.com/rheumatology/article-lookup/doi/10.1093/rheumatology/keq263

15 Margaretten M, Julian L, Katz P, Edward Yelin E. Depression in

patients with rheumatoid arthritis: Description, causes and mechanisms. Int J Clin Rheumtol. 2011 Dec 28 [cited 2017 Mar 22]; 6(6): 617–623. Available from: https://www.ncbi.nlm.nih.gov/pmc/articles/PMC3247620/

[16] Gibofsky A. Overview of epidemiology, pathophysiology, and diagnosis of rheumatoid arthritis. American Journal of Managed Care [website]. 2012 Dec 24 [cited 2017 Mar 22]. Available from: http://www.ajmc.com/journals/supplement/2012/ace006_12dec_ra/ace006_12dec_gibofsky_s295to302

[17] Doiron L. What are the different stages of rheumatoid arthritis? Conversant Bio [website]. 2014 Sep 9 [cited 2017 Mar 22]. Available from: http://www.conversantbio.com/blog/bid/396167/what-are-the-different-stages-of-rheumatoid-arthritis

[18] Hickson et al. Development of reduced kidney function in rheumatoid arthritis. (See footnote Chapter 6.)

[19] O'Dell JR, Mikuls TR. To improve outcomes we must define and measure them: Toward defining remission in rheumatoid arthritis. Arthritis Rheum. 2011 Mar [cited 2016 Mar 5];63(3):587–589. Available from: http://onlinelibrary.wiley.com/store/10.1002/art.30199/asset/30199_ftp.pdf?v=1&t=ilf64ghg&s=778909f43992c22affe8867dc5cf960bdec337df DOI:10.1002/art.30199

[20] Atzeni F, Antivalle M, Pallavicini FB, Caporali R, Bazzani C, Gorla R, Favalli EG, Marchesoni A, Sarzi-Puttini P. Predicting response to anti-TNF treatment in rheumatoid arthritis patients. Autoimmun Rev. 2009 Jan 27 [cited 2016 Mar 5]; 8(5):431-7. Available from: http://linkinghub.elsevier.com/retrieve/pii/S1568-9972(09)00009-3 DOI: 10.1016/j.autrev.2009

[21] Hetland ML, Christensen IJ, Tarp U, Dreyer L, Hansen A, Hansen IT, Kollerup G, Linde L, Lindegaard HM, Poulsen UE, et al. Direct

comparison of treatment responses, remission rates, and drug adherence in patients with rheumatoid arthritis treated with adalimumab, etanercept, or infliximab. Arthritis Rheum. 2010 Jan [cited 2016 Mar 5];62(1):22–32. Available from: http://onlinelibrary.wiley.com/doi/10.1002/art.27227/full DOI 10.1002/art.27227

[22] Singh et al. Biologics for rheumatoid arthritis. (See footnote Chapter 2.)

[23] Young K. A methotrexate alternative for rheumatoid arthritis? Rheumatoid Arthritis Warrior [website]. 2011 Aug 15 [cited 2016 Mar 5]. Available from: http://rawarrior.com/a-methotrexate-alternative-for-rheumatoid-arthritis/

[24] Young K. Efficacy of Xeljanz, biologics, & DMARDs in rheumatoid disease. Rheumatoid Arthritis Warrior [website]. 2013 May 13 [cited 2016 Mar 5]. Available from: http://rawarrior.com/efficacy-of-xeljanz-biologics-dmards-in-rheumatoid-disease/

[25] Lopez-Olivo MA, Siddhanamatha HR, Shea B, Tugwell P, Wells GA, Suarez-Almazor ME. Methotrexate for treating rheumatoid arthritis. The Cochrane Library [website]. 2014 Jun 2 [cited 2016 Mar 5]. Available from: http://onlinelibrary.wiley.com/o/cochrane/clabout/articles/MUSKEL/frame.html DOI: 10.1002/14651858.CD000957.pub2

[26] Grigor C, Capell H, Stirling A, McMahon AD, Lock P, Vallance R, Porter D. Effect of a treatment strategy of tight control for rheumatoid arthritis (the TICORA study): A single-blind randomised controlled trial. Lancet. 2004 [cited 2017 Mar 21];364:263-269. Available from: http://www.thelancet.com/journals/lancet/article/PIIS0140-6736(04)16676-2/fulltext

[27] Shahouri SH, Michaud K, Mikuls TR, Caplan L, Shaver TS, Anderson JD, Weidensaul DN, Busch RE, Wang S, Wolfe F.

Remission of rheumatoid arthritis in clinical practice: Application of the ACR/EULAR 2011 Remission Criteria. Arthritis Rheum. 2011 Nov [cited 2016 Mar 5];63(11): 3204–3215. Available from: http://www.ncbi.nlm.nih.gov/pmc/articles/PMC3202065/ DOI: 10.1002/art.30524

[28] Wolfe F. How am I doing? (See footnote Chapter 2.)

[29] Irvine S, Capell HC. Great expectations of modern RA treatment. Ann Rheum Dis. 2005 [cited 2016 Mar 5];64(9):1249-1251. Available from: http://ard.bmj.com/content/64/9/1249.full DOI:10.1136/ard.2005.039339

[30] Prince FHM, Bykerk VP, Shadick NA, Lu B, Cui J, Frits M, Iannaccone CK, Weinblatt ME, Solomon DH. Sustained rheumatoid arthritis remission is uncommon in clinical practice. Arthritis Res Ther. 2012 Mar 19 [cited 2016 Mar 5];14:R68 Available from: http://arthritis-research.biomedcentral.com/articles/10.1186/ar3785 DOI: 10.1186/ar3785

[31] Rindfleisch JA, Muller D. Diagnosis and management of rheumatoid arthritis. Am Fam Physician. 2005 Sep 15 [cited 2016 Mar 5];72(6):1037-1047. Available from: http://www.aafp.org/afp/2005/0915/p1037.html

[32] Smolen JS, Breedveld FC, Burmester GR, Bykerk V, Dougados M, Emery P, Kvien TK, Navarro-Compán MV, Oliver S, Schoels M, et al. Treating rheumatoid arthritis to target: 2014 update of the recommendations of an international task force. Ann Rheum Dis. 2015 May 12 [cited 2016 Mar 5];75:3 499-510. Available from: http://ard.bmj.com/content/early/2015/05/12/annrheumdis-2015-207524 DOI:10.1136/annrheumdis-2015-207524

[33] Irvine S. Great expectations. See footnote Chapter 8.)

[34] Pincus T, Tugwell P. Shouldn't standard rheumatology clinical care be evidence-based rather than eminence-based, eloquence-based, or

elegance-based? J Rheumatol. 2007 Jan [cited 2017 Mar 21];34(1): 1-4. Available from: http://www.jrheum.org/content/34/1/1.long

[35] Caceres V. ACR launches first public relations campaign. The Rheumatologist [Internet], 2011 Sep 1 [cited 2017 Mar 21]. Available from: http://www.the-rheumatologist.org/article/acr-launches-first-public-relations-campaign/

[36] Kavanagh R. The sexiness and cool of rheumatology. Personal blog, Wordpress [website]. 2011 Oct [cited 2011 Nov 2]. Available from: http://ronankavanagh.wordpress.com/2011/10/30/the-sexiness-and-cool-of-rheumatology/

[37] Pfizer, Inc. Tofacitinib for the treatment of rheumatoid arthritis, NDA 203214 [briefing document]. 2012 May 9 [cited 2013 Mar 23]. Available from Silver Spring (MD): Food and Drug Administration [website]. Available from: http://www.fda.gov/downloads/AdvisoryCommittees/CommitteesMeetingMaterials/Drugs/ArthritisAdvisoryCommittee/UCM302960.pdf

[38] Singh et al. Biologics for rheumatoid arthritis. (See footnote Chapter 2.)

[39] Young K. Efficacy of Xeljanz, Biologics, & DMARDs. (See footnote Chapter 8.)

[40] Young K. When rheumatology is sexy. Rheumatoid Arthritis Warrior [website]. 2011 Nov 2 [cited 2017 Mar 21]. Available from: http://rawarrior.com/when-rheumatology-is-sexy/

CHAPTER NINE
BETTER OUTCOMES
FOR PATIENTS

Acknowledging systemic disease aspects will improve medical outcomes.

Alleviating the mortality gap with RD

Recognition of the health dangers of RD can lead to more thorough care and improved outcomes. This recognition has gradually unfolded over several decades, and today many medical professionals remain unaware of its serious implications.

Mortality is a palpable example. For mortality outcomes to improve, clinicians must recognize the impact of systemic disease effects. Patients' lives depend on it. But the assessments of clinicians are based largely on their perceptions of the disease, as the following examples illustrate.

Writing in 1991, Stanford University's Edward Harris described a contemporary study spanning 25 years that found "Rheumatoid disease (including vasculitis)" to be cause the of death in 19 percent of patients, and "in a further 14% RA was a contributory factor. These data conform with numerous other surveys published in the past 40 years."[1] Thus, Harris found

RD to be either a cause or a contributory factor to death in 33% of patients.

Harris found CVD was the cause of death in 46 percent of the patients, infection in 17%, and malignancy in 13%. However, if he were writing in 2017, there might be greater recognition of the impact of RD on each of these causes of death, as he obviously noted with vasculitis. Cause of death for infection in people with RD (PRD) was later recognized to be 9%, versus 1% in the general population.[2] In recent years malignancy has also shown to be increased as a result of RD. (For more on CVD in RD, see Chapter 5.)

Another report, in 1999, challenged numerous other studies that had shown the standard mortality ratio (SMR) is increased in RA.[3] (SMR lower than 100 reflects less mortality than the general population; SMR over 100 shows higher mortality.) Lindqvist reported an "SMR of 87 ...in contrast with previous studies where SMR varied from 130 in a population based study of Pima Indians in Arizona to 300 in a hospital based study from Birmingham." In Lindqvist's study, 18 of 183 patients died, and the authors concluded, "No RA related variable contributed significantly to an increased risk of death."

However, examination of actual causes of death (in the study's Table 3) reveals that nine of the 18 died of cardiovascular causes, one of alcoholism, one of infection, and seven of malignancy. Of the cancer-related deaths, one was a postoperative infection and two were bronchial carcinoma. Two deaths were complicated, with RA considered to be a possible contributor. A re-examination of the deaths in this small study, with consideration of subsequently established systemic aspects of RD, especially CVD, might lead to a different conclusion about SMR.

If "RA" is understood to be arthritis or joint inflammation, its prospective impact on mortality may not be recognized. However, if RD is recognized as the dangerous disease that this book demonstrates it to be, its impact on serious health problems or on mortality is understood differently. What a doctor expects of a disease can affect how she views both SMR data and the patient in front of her.

In 2002, a study over six times as large as Lindqvist's (>1,200 patients) found excess mortality in early inflammatory polyarthritis "confined to patients who are seropositive for RF (rheumatoid factor). While excess cardiovascular mortality has been described in patients with established RA, this is the first report of premature death from heart disease in the early years of IP (inflammatory polyarthritis)."[4] Likely, though the arthritis was not yet well established in those patients, *the rheumatoid disease was*. Goodson et al. concluded that it would be beneficial for clinicians to know of the increased risk and be able to identify patients with such risks: "The ability to identify patients at increased risk of death from cardiovascular causes is obviously of interest to the clinician." Further, Goodson acknowledged it remains to be proven whether aggressive disease control or targeted modification of CVD risk factors "or a combination of the two would actually reduce cardiovascular mortality rates in the seropositive RA."

A recent French study, ten times the size of Goodson's, assessed over 13,000 deaths related to RA in an epidemiological database spanning eleven years.[5] Avouac et al. found that, in 4,597 cases, RA was the underlying cause of death (UCD) and in 8,611 cases, RA was an associated cause of death (ACD). Their analysis was very detailed and obviously influenced by recognition of current knowledge of the associations of RD with each health threat. They conclude: "These data support the need to expand new strategies to prevent infectious and cardiovascular diseases in order to improve survival of RA patients."[6]

Patients and doctors both must know the dangers of RD

One pulmonary symptom of rheumatoid disease, fibrosing alveolitis (FA), provides a clear example of the need for both clinicians and patients to know more about the various effects of RD, and to be aware of common risks even in people who may seem asymptomatic. Dawson wrote that FA is considered "both the most common and most serious pleuropulmonary complication of RA;"[7] but, "(t)he literature on FA in patients with RA is confusing and varies from series to series, depending on diagnostic criteria." A study population consisting of 150 consecutive RA patients, selected irrespective of chest symptoms or signs, found 28 suffered from FA (19%).

Clinicians should be educated to suspect FA in PRD with shortness of breath (dyspnea) and order appropriate tests or refer to a suitable specialist: "HRCT evidence of FA was present in 19% of hospital outpatients with RA. Abnormalities on chest examination or on full pulmonary function tests, even without restrictive changes or chest radiographic abnormalities, should prompt physicians to request a chest HRCT scan when investigating dyspnoea in patients with RA." Dawson also found 28 patients had thickened interlobular lines; 23 had emphysematous bullae; and there were numerous other abnormalities detected in the patients' lungs as shown in Table 2 of the report.

Many of the patients discussed by Dawson would likely not know of their status with regard to FA or the numerous other lung abnormalities had they not been part of a clinical study. Lung problems are not something that is looked for in PRD.

Well-meaning and otherwise well-educated people are simply unaware of the effect of RD on the lungs. Meanwhile investigators of lungs and other organs are recommending a higher level of scrutiny in PRD: "Given the prevalence of lung involvement in RA, clinicians should have a low threshold to pursue evaluation of new respiratory complaints in this population."[8] We must take steps to make patients and clinicians both aware that the disease affects the lungs and other organs. See Chapter 13 for how you can help.

Challenging conventional notions and methods can improve outcomes

Therefore, the distinction between "rheumatoid arthritis" and "rheumatoid disease" is one with real differences. Arthritis unavoidably connotes joint inflammation, necessitating awkward use of words such as "complication" or "comorbidity" to describe extra-articular aspects of the disease like FA or CVD. A decade ago, experts indicated that "traditional measures of RA disease activity may not necessarily be the best predictors of mortality"[9] in rheumatoid patients. As long as those traditional measures (rheumatoid factor, radiographic erosion of joints, and musculoskeletal pain) are the principal methods to assess rheumatoid disease, that excess mortality cannot be adequately addressed. The same experts advise that the "undertreatment of comorbidity, especially cardiovascular comorbidity, and underlying risk factors is a matter of concern to all rheumatologists." *Addressing that undertreatment will necessarily improve outcomes.*

Scientific investigation of how rheumatoid disease activity causes FA, CVD, and other contributors to RD mortality will help reverse outdated notions like blaming medications or patients' lack of ability to exercise for all excess mortality. As discussed in Chapter 5, examination of the mechanisms of CVD in RD has increased, for example. One NIH grant titled "Mechanisms Linking Joint Inflammation and Atherosclerosis in Rheumatoid Arthritis" is examining the effect of disease activity on lipoprotein function.[10] Other studies mentioned earlier explore the relationship between RD-specific antibodies and remodeling of the left ventricle of the heart (Chapter 3) or between high disease activity and higher mortality risk (Chapter 6). Investigators are even attempting to create a study model of the disease that includes the "greater atherosclerotic burden" of RD.[11]

The support of several such investigations with public and private funding of tens of millions of dollars demonstrates that, at least in part, the scientific community recognizes the health threats posed by RD. NIH-funded researcher Christina Charles-Schoeman explains why these investigations are essential: "Cardiovascular disease (CVD) is the leading killer of patients with rheumatoid arthritis (RA) who have a 2-3 fold increased risk of myocardial infarction compared to members of the general population. Traditional cardiovascular (CV) risk factors alone do not accurately predict CVD in RA patients and therefore adequate primary prevention strategies are lacking."[12]

SOLVING THESE 3 PROBLEMS CAN IMPROVE CARE NOW

Undertreatment is a result of the murky perception of the disease on the part of everyone involved in RD care, including patients. Solving these three problems would generate dramatic improvement similar to the improvement in diabetes care in recent decades.

PROBLEM ONE: People with RD do not receive appropriate preventive care.

People with RD are less likely to receive preventive care than other patients, and less likely than other chronic disease patients.[13, 14] In a population where preventive services are even more critical, fewer are performed. According to Gabriel, "Such services include blood pressure testing, lipids profile testing, flu vaccination, pneumococcal vaccination, mammograms and cervical cancer screening. We showed that patients with RA do not receive optimal health maintenance and preventive care services. Davis and colleagues also showed that *patients with RA with a clinical diagnosis of heart failure were less likely to undergo echocardiography and less likely to be prescribed cardiovascular drugs*—for example, ACE inhibitors, β blockers and diuretics."[15]

Kremers, et al. investigated areas of preventive care that relate to three main causes of mortality in PRD.[16] With regard to these three, they found: "Patients with RA do not receive optimal health maintenance and preventive care services. Efforts should be made, on the part of all physicians who care for RA patients, to ensure that these effective preventive services are provided."

- Cardiovascular disease – lipid profile, blood pressure testing

- Malignancies – mammogram, Papanicolaou smears

- Infection – vaccinations for flu or pneumonia

The urgency for preventive care has been underscored by a few researchers, but the problem remains. Obviously, the notion of what constitutes care for "rheumatoid arthritis" must be adjusted.

PROBLEM TWO: Guidelines and tools are insufficient, and are not followed.

As with diagnostic criteria (discussed in Chapter 3), RA care guidelines do not incorporate assessment or treatment of systemic aspects of the disease (discussed in Chapters 5 and 6).[17, 18, 19] Even when partial recommendations are in place (e.g. for pneumonia vaccination or tuberculosis testing prior to biologic treatment), third party payers (insurance or government) do not consider them essential to be performed and may refuse to accept costs, despite whether similar care would be allowed for more well-known disease populations.

PRD are not typically referred for cardiovascular evaluations and traditional methods for assessing cardiovascular risk, the Framingham Risk Score and Reynolds Risk Score, are inadequate to estimate risk in PRD. In 2009, the European League Against Rheumatism published recommendations for estimating CVD risk in RA, which, if fully developed and put into practice, could be a good step for European patients.[20]

For rheumatoid lung disease, "no consensus therapeutic guidelines have been established" because, according to Yunt, no therapeutic trials have been performed."[21] The same is true for most of the health dangers discussed in this book.

Rheumatology should implement strategies that move closer to a holistic therapeutic paradigm and take advantage of the latest knowledge about pre-RA. Scottish doctor Iain McInnes pronounces these as "exciting times for rheumatologists."[22] These new leads make imminent a quantum leap in the care and prevention or delay of onset of full-blown disease. But rheumatology must take advantage of them.

PROBLEM THREE: An annual review is not conducted.

An adequate annual review is possibly the single most significant way to advance comprehensive care for PRD. In *What kills patients with rheumatoid arthritis?* Kelly and

Hamilton suggested in 2007, "Perhaps rheumatologists should consider revising the approach adopted in the routine assessment of RA patients by using an annual review form to include the systemic aspects of the disease in addition to its articular manifestations. This could be roughly analogous to the approach taken by diabetologists for decades, which has helped to reduce mortality through regularly recording of predictors such as blood lipid profiles, blood pressure, hepatic and renal function, together with a global measurement of disease activity."[23]

Such an annual review should provide opportunity for appropriate consideration of common extra-articular aspects of RD, with realistic recommendations for addressing risks. This may necessitate development of tools that help patients and clinicians decide what tests should be performed to help identify what steps should be taken to preserve the health of a particular patient. Tools to aid diagnosis, monitor disease activity, and make treatment decisions should take into account common features of systemic disease such as those discussed in this book. Having such tools in place would strengthen the ability of doctors to improve outcomes of PRD.

The following essay is adapted from an article on rawarrior.com[24]

WHAT IF ONLY THE CANCER IN DAVE'S KIDNEYS WAS TREATED?

Measuring disease activity: where rubber meets the road

Recently a rheumatologist friend told me of needing to prove ACR20 (a measure of 20 percent improvement) to insurance in order for a patient to continue receiving a biologic treatment. I don't know whether it was private or government insurance, but something bothered me about it.

Of course, 20 percent improvement (ACR20) is not very dramatic. A friend in the pharmaceutical industry once asked me, "Would your life be much better if we could treat four of your twenty inflamed joints?"

In this case, what concerned me was something else. ACR20 (supposedly reserved for clinical trials) measures improvement *of musculoskeletal symptoms*. The same is true for all six of ACR's recently recommended measures of disease activity: CDAI, DAS28 (with ESR or CRP), PAS, PAS-II, RAPID-3, and SDAI.[25] (ESR and CRP may provide systemic signs in some patients; and a patient "global assessment" is a small part of each formula, but that is generally stated in terms of "your arthritis.")

Measuring beyond synovitis? And beyond joints?

Attention is not given to symptoms beyond joints—or often even beyond synovitis (inflamed synovial tissue). What if a person's joint symptoms did not improve enough, but his lung symptoms did? I know a person like this whose rheumatoid lung disease was brought under control by methotrexate, while joint symptoms continued. Of course the opposite scenario is equally troublesome, and probably more common: a person's synovitis improving, with little or no attention paid to non-articular aspects of the disease.

Some patients receive medical attention for extra-articular (outside of joint) symptoms of rheumatoid disease and many do not. Either way, I've never heard of including them in a measure of disease activity. And that makes sense because those symptoms are not tracked or treated by rheumatologists.

Rheumatologists are trained to identify and evaluate rheumatic diseases by particular musculoskeletal symptoms (although there are often discrepancies there as well).[26]

So-called "arthritis" in the eyes

Last year, I read the story of Sandy Blue on Mayo Clinic's blog.[27] Of course it's impossible to have joint inflammation ("arthritis") in the eyes since there are no joints in the eyes. Sandy saw eight eye specialists over six months before finally traveling to Mayo Clinic where a "team approach" allowed her to be diagnosed with Rheumatoid Arthritis. Sandy's first apparent symptom of RA was her scleritis, which inflamed her eyes so badly she could not see.

Not an aberration

It's not uncommon for the first or the worst symptoms of rheumatoid disease to be extra-articular. It's a possibility you've read in several observations from investigators quoted in this book. And I'll never forget the first time (in 2009) I asked people about their very first rheumatoid symptoms.[28] Or the wide variety of responses such as Andrew's:

"My first symptoms were iritis (inflammation) in eyes, then ankle problems (torn Achilles tendons resulting in surgery on both sides). Not until extreme fatigue hit me last year coupled with finger swelling and pain did I get diagnosed with RA and start on treatment. While my symptoms did eventually spread to all fingers, wrists, elbows, and knees (my latest big battle), it all started with 'non typical' RA symptoms that didn't meet the traditional RA patterns."

If you work in the healthcare industry, especially if you're a clinician who treats people with RD, I hope you'll take advantage of the 880 responses to that article. While it may be impossible to determine a frequency of occurrence of each initial symptom, the list does reflect the wide range of symptoms that patients report. (See list in Chapter 1.) *I'm not sure I've ever met a patient who experiences only synovitis, so my guess is they are rare.*

Can the lack of a comprehensive grasp of RA harm patients?

If you're a caregiver or patient, questions or difficulties you've encountered in treating this disease are usually related to this problem—including a need for more effective drugs. How can drug developers find solutions when the problem is so ill defined? Does it matter if symptoms related to the disease are not recorded in the chart of the rheumatologist? **Yes, in more ways than I can count in one post.**

What if they'd only treated the kidneys in e-Patient Dave's stage IV renal cell carcinoma, (described in his book *Laugh, Sing, and Eat Like a Pig: How an Empowered Patient Beat Stage IV Cancer (and what healthcare can learn from it)*) instead of all the sites it affected him?[29] You would not treat a patient's metastatic kidney cancer only in his kidneys if it has spread to the rest of his body. It should be the same with RD— you must treat every aspect of the disease.

The change that patients need

1. We need healthcare professionals to have a clearer more complete understanding of this disease.
2. We need more suitable measurement tools and diagnostic criteria.
3. We need medical care that is more comprehensive in its approach.
4. We obviously need a better name for a disease that's

not "a type of arthritis."

Of course, adding the patient voice is the way to improve care AND research related to rheumatoid disease. Whether you're a patient or provide any kind of care or benefit to rheumatoid patients, I hope you'll stand with patients by joining the Rheumatoid Patient Foundation at rheum4us.org.

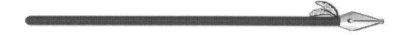

KEY POINTS

1. As we learn more about extra-articular disease, we see more clearly the impact on RD mortality.

2. Patients and clinicians must both become aware of the extra-articular effects of RD.

3. Experts acknowledge that traditional measures of RA are not the best predictors of mortality.

4. Investigators are searching for specific ways disease activity causes extra-articular disease or contributes to mortality.

5. Steps to improve care:

   a) PRD need appropriate preventive care.

   b) Improve diagnostic criteria and treatment guidelines to correspond to current knowledge of RD.

   c) Conduct annual reviews of systemic disease in all PRD.

Action step: Combat excess mortality in RD by conducting annual reviews of systemic disease activity.

Quote to remember: If "RA" is understood to be arthritis or joint inflammation, its prospective impact on mortality may not be recognized. However, if RD is recognized as the dangerous disease that this book demonstrates it to be, its impact on serious health problems or on mortality is understood differently. What a doctor expects of a disease can affect how she views both SMR data and the patient in front of her.

---

[1] Harris, ED. Pathogenesis of rheumatoid arthritis: Its relevance to therapy in the '90s. Trans Am Clin Climatol Assoc. 1991 [cited 2013 Jun 21];102:260–270. Available from: http://www.ncbi.nlm.nih.gov/pmc/articles/PMC2376656/

[2] Boers et al. Making an impact on mortality in rheumatoid arthritis. (See footnote Chapter 3.)

[3] Lindqvist E, Eberhardt K. Mortality in rheumatoid arthritis patients with disease in the 1980s. Ann Rheum Dis. 1999 [cited 2013 Jun 22]; 58:1-14. Available from: http://ard.bmj.com/content/58/1/11.full

[4] Goodson NJ, Wiles NJ, Lunt M, Barrett EM, Silman A, Symmons DPM. Mortality in early inflammatory polyarthritis. Arthritis Rheum. 2002 Aug [cited 2013 Jun 21];46:2010-9. Available from: http://onlinelibrary.wiley.com/doi/10.1002/art.10419/full

[5] Avouac J, Amrouche F, Meune C, Rey G, Kahan A, Allanore Y. Mortality profile of patients with rheumatoid arthritis in France and its change in 10 years. Semin Arthritis Rheum. 2016 Oct 29 [cited 2017 Jul 9];46(5),537-543. Available from: http://www.semarthritisrheumatism.com/article/S0049-0172(16)30372-9/fulltext

[6] Avouac et al. Mortality profile of patients with rheumatoid arthritis in France. (See footnote Chapter 9.)

[7] Dawson JK, Fewins HE, Desmond J, Lynch MP, Graham DR. Fibrosing alveolitis in patients with rheumatoid arthritis as assessed by high resolution computed tomography, chest radiography and pulmonary function tests. Thorax. 2001 [cited 2013 Jun 21]; 56:622-7. Available from: http://thorax.bmj.com/content/56/8/622.full

[8] Yunt ZX. Lung disease in rheumatoid arthritis. (See footnote Chapter 2.)

[9] Boers et al. Making an impact on mortality in rheumatoid arthritis. (See footnote Chapter 3.)

[10] National Institutes of Health [website]. NIH research grant 5R01HL123064-02 displayed in Estimates of Funding for Various Research, Condition, and Disease Categories. 2017 Jul 2 [cited 2017 Aug 1] Available from: https://report.nih.gov/categorical_spending.aspx

[11] National Institutes of Health [website]. NIH research grant 4R01AR064546-04 displayed in Estimates of Funding for Various Research, Condition, and Disease Categories. 2017 Jul 2 [cited 2017 Aug 1] Available from: https://report.nih.gov/categorical_spending.aspx

[12] National Institutes of Health [website]. NIH research grant 5R01HL123064-02. (See footnote chapter 9.)

[13] Musculoskeletal Network [website]. Cardiovascular risk in RA patients: Falling between the cracks? 2013 Feb 8 [cited 2013 Feb 14]. Available from: http://www.rheumatologynetwork.com/articles/cardiovascular-risk-ra-patients-falling-between-cracks

[14] Young K. Problems with preventive care and rheumatoid arthritis

mortality. Rheumatoid Arthritis Warrior [website]. 2010 Aug 20[cited 2017 Mar 22]. Available from: http://rawarrior.com/ problems-with-preventive-care-and-rheumatoid-arthritis-mortality/

[15] Gabriel SE. Why do people with rheumatoid arthritis still die prematurely? (See footnote in Chapter 1.)

[16] Kremers HM, Bidaut-Russell M, Scott CG, Reinalda MS, Zinsmeister AR, Gabriel SE. Preventive medical services among patients with rheumatoid arthritis. J Rheumatol. 2003 Sep [cited 2013 Mar 23];30(9):1940-1947. Available from: http:// www.jrheum.org/content/30/9/1940.long

[17] Saag KG, Yazdany J, Alexander C, Caplan L, Coblyn J, Desai Sp, Harrington T, Liu J, Mcniff K, Newman E, et al. Defining quality of care in rheumatology: The American College of Rheumatology white paper on quality measurement. Arthrit Care Res. 2011 Jan [cited 2013 Mar 23];63(1):2–9. DOI 10.1002/acr.20369

[18] Yazdany J, MacLean CH. Quality of care in the rheumatic diseases: Current status and future directions. Curr Opin Rheumatol. 2008 Mar [cited 2017 Mar 21];20(2):159-66

[19] Harrold LR, Harrington JT, Curtis JR, Furst DE, Bentley MJ, Shan Y, Reed G, Kremer J, Greenberg JD. Prescribing practices in a US cohort of rheumatoid arthritis patients before and after publication of the American College of Rheumatology treatment recommendations. Arthritis Rheum. 2012 Mar [cited 2017 Mar 21]; 64(3):630–638. Available from: http://onlinelibrary.wiley.com/doi/ 10.1002/art.33380/full

[20] Peters et al. EULAR evidence-based recommendations for cardiovascular risk. (See footnote Chapter 8.)

[21] Yunt ZX. Lung disease in rheumatoid arthritis. (See footnote Chapter 2.)

[22] McInnes IB. Nine gaps in our understanding of RA: Openings to yet better outcomes. Rheumatology Network [website]. 2013 May 20 [cited 2017 Mar 22]. Available from: http://www.rheumatologynetwork.com/articles/nine-gaps-our-understanding-ra-openings-yet-better-outcomes

[23] Kelly C, Hamilton J. What kills patients with rheumatoid arthritis? (See footnote Chapter 5.)

[24] Young K. Where the rubber meets the road or what if only the cancer in Dave's kidneys was treated? Rheumatoid Arthritis Warrior. [website]. 2013 Mar 11 [cited 2013 Jun 30]. Available from: http://rawarrior.com/where-the-rubber-meets-the-road-or-what-if-only-the-cancer-in-daves-kidneys-was-treated/

[25] Anderson J, Caplan L, et al. Rheumatoid arthritis disease activity measures. (See footnote Chapter 5.)

[26] Young K. Disparity between rheumatoid arthritis patients & doctors over disease activity. Rheumatoid Arthritis Warrior [website]. 2012 Aug 3 [cited 2013 Jun 30]. Available from: http://rawarrior.com/disparity-between-rheumatoid-arthritis-patients-doctors-over-disease-activity/

[27] Rivas R. Rare arthritis no match for woman determined to save her eyesight. (See footnote Chapter 4.)

[28] Young K. What is the first symptom of rheumatoid arthritis? (See footnote Chapter 4.)

[29] deBronkart RD. Laugh, sing, and eat like a pig: How an empowered patient beat stage IV cancer (and what healthcare can learn from it). Media, PA: Changing Outlook Press; 2010. 260 p.

CHAPTER TEN
BENEFICIAL DISEASE NAME CHANGES

Here are six examples of improved outcomes that resulted from updating disease names.

Names evolve with knowledge

The evolution of other disease names provides insight into both the wisdom and the means for making such purposeful changes. Numerous conditions have been re-named for a variety of reasons, but we look at six that particularly inform us.

ONE: From Reiter's Syndrome to Reactive Arthritis

The substitution of "reactive arthritis" for "Reiter's syndrome" has been voluntary and gradual. Although there was a worthy reason for the change, the process has unfortunately been incomplete and imprecise.

Reactive arthritis (ReA) is a rare disease that can occur as an acute episode (lasting less than six months) or continue as a chronic condition with recurring bouts of symptoms. Today ReA is considered a seronegative spondyloarthropathy, with a serologically negative rheumatic factor and often a positive HLA-B27 (referring the gene called human leukocyte antigen).

ReA is believed to be triggered by a bacterial infection (enteric or urogenital).[1]

The case of ReA is of particular interest because of two things it has in common with rheumatoid disease: 1) It is rheumatological condition with 2) a historical backdrop. According to forensic historians, Christopher Columbus suffered from ReA, acquired via a food-borne infection.[2]

ReA was first referred to as "Reiter's disease" in 1942 by two authors relying heavily upon a description of a syndrome described by Hans Reiter in 1916 that involved arthritis, conjunctivitis, and urethritis.[3, 4] The authors may not have been aware of reports by numerous other investigators who described similar patients. Some of these reports date back as early as 1776, according to Matteson, et.al.

The term Reiter's syndrome was commonly used until its namesake, Hans Reiter, became widely known as a National Socialist (Nazi) war criminal. As Reiter's avid support of Hitler's Third Reich grew in the general consciousness, many had a strong aversion to the eponym's use. In "Why Change the Name of Reiter's Syndrome?" Matteson, et al. argues for a rejection of the eponym *Reiter's* and for a change in name for this. condition.[5] They cite historical evidence that Hans Reiter participated in Nazi experiments resulting in hundreds of deaths and that he supported the National Socialist Workers' Party as early as 1931.

Consequently, use of Reiter's name has declined; however, it has not been completely abandoned. For some patients, continued use of the reference is a point of concern. Yet, the term *reactive arthritis* is not perfectly synonymous with *Reiter's syndrome*. The original syndrome is more than arthritis; it is a triad of symptoms: arthritis, conjunctivitis, and urethritis. Furthermore, it may have serous extra articular manifestations[6] including cardiac symptoms thought to have been responsible for the death of Columbus. *Reactive arthritis* is not adequate since it expressly refers to joint inflammation as a consequence of infection. However, the word "arthritis" seems to have stuck, meaning that patients are left with a term that even Matteson agrees is insufficient.

TWO: From Gay-related Immune Deficiency (or Gay cluster disease) to Acquired Immune Deficiency Syndrome (AIDS) and Human Immunodeficiency Virus (HIV)

A name for the disease and the virus that causes it were necessary steps toward successful research that led to treatment.

During the first years of AIDS treatment and research, a cloud of fear and misinformation hovered over the nameless disease. In the early 1980's AIDS was referred to in several ways including GRID (gay-related immune deficiency)[7] and "4H" disease (referring to homosexuals, hemophiliacs, heroin users, and Haitians).[8]

In September of 1982, the CDC adopted the name ***acquired immune deficiency syndrome*** (AIDS).[9] In 1986, the actual virus finally acquired its own name ***human immunodeficiency virus*** (HIV) at a World Health Organization meeting in Paris, where warnings were also given about how many people might be infected. Subsequent research led to dramatic improvements in outcomes and treatments.[10]

THREE: From Wegener's Granulomatosis to Granulomatosis with Polyangiitis (GPA) or

(Vasculitis)

This recent and fascinating name-change story involves, once again, a rare rheumatological disease, the Nazi's, and the research of Mayo Clinic's Dr. Eric Matteson.[11] In this case, the name change was deliberate.

Wegener's granulomatosis is a rare disease in which blood vessels become inflamed. The American College of Rheumatology[12] estimates it affects 3 out of every 100,000 people. Estimates of annual incidence are between 8 and 9 per 1 million people.[13] Recent discoveries about the extent of Friedrich Wegener's involvement with the Nazi regime prompted a movement in the medical community to remove his eponym[14] and rebrand the disease as **granulomatosis with polyangiitis** (GPA).

Although the change was initiated by medical professionals, it was complicated. "The efforts to rename this disease process have been stifled given the universal acceptance in medical literature of the term Wegener's granulomatosis describing the well known vasculitic syndrome."[15]

Since GPA is a type of vasculitis, a decision was also made to change the name of the Wegener's Granulomatosis Association (WGA) to the Vasculitis Foundation (VF). This effort was also met with resistance, this time from patients. Some patient communities and blogs pushed back.[16] In 2006, Dr. Gary Hoffman responded by outlining reasons for the change:

"Most of our members have supported the name change from the Wegener's Granulomatosis Association (WGA) to the Vasculitis Foundation (VF). Others have felt a trust had been betrayed. Explanations were offered to try to convey the scientific and organizational logic for the change. Still, unfortunately, not everyone has "gotten it". In this article, we will try to make the reasons for change as clear as possible and hope that all of our readers will become better informed and most importantly satisfied that this is not only the right thing to do, but also the only logical course to follow."[17]

Dr. Hoffman discusses reasons for a name change, each of which is familiar to people with rheumatoid disease:

- Establish medical accuracy

- Provide a wider scope of research focus

- Increase the minimal NIH research funding

- Enable all vasculitis patients to advocate together for better research and treatments

- Consider childhood forms of the disease

FOUR: From Lou Gehrig's Disease to Amyotrophic Lateral Sclerosis (ALS)

This has been a gradual change that embraces both terms. Adoption of the scientific term has had a two-fold effect. It has both improved public awareness about the nature of the disease and encouraged more research.

Amyotrophic lateral sclerosis or ALS is extremely rare; as few as 2 of every 100,000 people are diagnosed with it. For many years, ALS was known in the U.S. as ***Lou Gehrig's disease***, after New York Yankees baseball player Lou Gehrig. However, the condition has had various labels in other countries. The British and Australians say ***motor neuron disease*** (MND) and the French say ***maladie de Charcot***. The renowned French neurologist Jean-Martin Charcot first described ALS in 1869.

Lou Gehrig's disease, the common term used in the U.S., has not been rejected, probably because it has made the public more aware of the disease. The ALS Association not only features a photograph of Lou Gehrig on the front page of its website, it also displays "Fighting Lou Gehrig's Disease" within its logo.[18] The ALS Association gratefully takes full advantage of their most famous patient who brought worldwide attention to this disease when he was forced to suddenly retire from baseball after being diagnosed.

FIVE: From Manic Depression to Bipolar Disorder

The new term is more accurate and descriptive of the extremes of mood experienced by patients. It has helped with disease stigma that resulted from a name that seemed to vilify patients.

Bipolar disorder is a mood disorder causing drastic mood changes "from manic, restless highs to depressive, listless lows," with alternating, episodic changes.[19] In 1980, the American Psychiatric Association updated its Diagnostic and Statistical Manual to re-label **manic depression** as bipolar disorder. This name change was the culmination of a gradual recognition of the insulting connotation of the previous designation. "Manic" sounds similar to "maniac" and seems to imply that psychotic episodes are common, when they actually rare.[20]

However, the disorder has a long history of unconstructive terminology, having been once termed "circular insanity" (Jules Falret, 1854).[21] Previously, this disorder has also been called *bipolar affective disorder* and *manic-depressive illness*. Experts say the modern term is more correct, encouraging better understanding of what patients experience.

SIX: From Huntington's Chorea to Huntington's Disease

Naming a devastating brain disease after only one of its symptoms was not advantageous to patients or researchers.

The disease is named for George Huntington who provided the first thorough description of the disease in 1872. The term **chorea** refers to uncontrolled movements that are a common observable symptom. However, according to the widow of one **Huntington's disease** (HD) patient, patients and family members are much more devastated by other aspects of the disease:

"The change from chorea to disease was made to reflect Huntington's is a far more complex disease than at first thought. Chorea is only one aspect and the focus has shifted over the years to the neurological changes affecting emotions; mood changes; obsessive compulsion; cognitive difficulties; loss of reasoning; motor degeneration and a whole host of other complex symptoms."[22]

MedicineNet agrees that the name was changed to better "describe this highly complex disorder that causes untold suffering for thousands of families."[23] An estimated 15,000 Americans have HD, a highly hereditary disease for which a single genetic defect is believed to be the cause. In 1968 the Hereditary Disease Foundation "was involved in the recruitment of over 100 scientists in the Huntington's Disease Collaborative Research Project who over a 10 year period worked to locate the responsible gene."[24]

In progress: Improving cancer treatment by updating terminology

A broad change in nomenclature has already begun in cancer to address the problem of overtreatment due to fear. The reasoning is parallel to changes needed in RD, correcting historical stereotypes. However, in RD, the problem is undertreatment, rather than overtreatment.

The National Cancer Institute has recommended that cancer terminology be changed based on "companion diagnostics" so that the word "cancer" would not be used in pre-malignant conditions or when potential malignancy risk is low.[25] Many patients and doctors agree that "hundreds of thousands of men and women are undergoing needless and sometimes disfiguring and harmful treatments for premalignant and cancerous lesions that are so slow growing they are unlikely to ever cause harm."[26]

Like other conditions that have required updated names, cancer suffers from historical stereotypes that conflict with modern research. According to Dr. Otis W. Brawley, chief medical officer for the American Cancer Society, "We need a 21st-century definition of cancer instead of a 19th-century definition of cancer, which is what we've been using."[27]

Name changes are ordinary and necessary

There are other examples of disease name changes beyond those described in this chapter. However, the six changes above and the current changes being sought in cancer terminology demonstrate that vocabulary changes are an ordinary part of the evolution of medicine. Name changes of diseases will always be necessary as medicine evolves and knowledge increases. Updating "rheumatoid arthritis" to "rheumatoid disease" is the natural step that follows the revelation that arthritis is only one symptom of a complex disease.

[1] Sarani N. Reactive arthritis in emergency medicine. Medscape Reference [website]. 2012 May 21 [cited 2012 Jul 21]. Available from: http://emedicine.medscape.com/article/808833-overview#a0104

[2] Young K. What kind of arthritis did Christopher Columbus have? Rheumatoid Arthritis Warrior [website]. 2009 Oct 13 [cited 2012 Jul 21]. Available from: http://rawarrior.com/what-kind-of-arthritis-did-christopher-columbus-have/

[3] Iglesias-Gammara A, Restrepo JF, Valle R, Matteson EL. A brief history of Stoll-Brodie-Fiessinger-Leroy syndrome (Reiter's syndrome) and reactive arthritis with a translation of Reiter's original 1916 article into English. Curr Rheumatol Rev. 2005 [cited 2012 Jul 20];1:71-79. Available from: http://www.benthamscience.com/crr/sample/crr1-1/D0011R.pdf

[4] Wikipedia contributors. Reactive arthritis. Wikipedia, The Free Encyclopedia [Internet]. 2013 Mar 8, [cited 2012 Jul 20]. Available from: http://en.wikipedia.org/wiki/Reactive_arthritis

[5] Iglesias-Gammara A. A brief history. (See footnote Chapter 10.)

[6] Iglesias-Gammara A. A brief history. (See footnote Chapter 10.)

[7] Wikipedia contributors. Gay-related immune deficiency. Wikipedia, The Free Encyclopedia [Internet]. 2013 Mar 5 [cited 2012 Jul 20]. Available from: http://en.wikipedia.org/wiki/Gay-related_immune_deficiency

[8] Wikipedia contributors. History of HIV/AIDS. Wikipedia, The Free Encyclopedia [Internet]. 2017 Oct 16 [cited 2017 Oct 21]. Available from: https://en.wikipedia.org/w/index.php?title=History_of_HIV/AIDS&oldid=805554235

[9] MMWR Weekly [Internet]. Current trends update on acquired

immune deficiency syndrome (AIDS) — United States. 1982 Sep 24 [cited 2012 July 21];31(37):507-508, 513-514. Available from: http://www.cdc.gov/mmwr/preview/mmwrhtml/00001163.htm

[10] Fischl MA, Richman DD, Grieco MH, Gottlieb MS, Volberding PA, Laskin OL, Leedom JM, Groopman JE, Mildvan D, Schooley RT, et al. The efficacy of azidothymidine (AZT) in the treatment of patients with AIDS and AIDS-related complex, a double-blind, placebo-controlled trial. New Engl J Med. 1987 Jul 23 [cited 2012 Jul 21]; 317(4):185-91. Available from: http://www.nejm.org/doi/full/ 10.1056/NEJM198707233170401 DOI:10.1056/ NEJM198707233170401

[11] Benson L. Mayo doctor helped spearhead name change for disorder with Nazi namesake. Minnesota Public Radio News [website]. 2011 May 18 [cited 2012 Jul 21]. Available from: http:// minnesota.publicradio.org/display/web/2011/05/18/nazi-named-disorder-name-change/

[12] American College of Rheumatology [website]. Granulomatosis with polyangiitis (Wegener's). 2011 Apr 10 [cited 2016 Mar 5]. Available from: http://www.rheumatology.org/I-Am-A/Patient-Caregiver/ Diseases-Conditions/Granulomatosis-with-Polyangitis-Wegners

[13] Watts RA, Al-Taiar A, Scott DG, Macgregor AJ. Prevalence and incidence of Wegener's granulomatosis in the UK general practice research database. Arthrit Car Res. 2009 Oct 15 [cited 2016 Mar 5]; 61(10):1412-1416. Available from: http://onlinelibrary.wiley.com/ doi/10.1002/art.24544/full

[14] Mora B, Bosch X. Medical eponyms: Time for a change. Arch Intern Med. 2010 [cited 2012 Jul 21];170(16):1499-1500. Available from: http://archinte.jamanetwork.com/article.aspx?articleid=225874 DOI:10.1001/archinternmed.2010.281

[15] Matoo, A. Grand Rounds: "ANCA-Associated Vasculitis: Update for

internists." Clinical Correlations [website]. New York University; 2008 Apr 9 [cited 2012 Jul 20]. Available from: http:// www.clinicalcorrelations.org/?p=699

[16] Bagley C. Name change of Wegner's granulomatosis. Sierra Sage [website]. 2011 Jun 3 [cited 2016 Mar 5]. Available from: https:// cynbagleymedical.wordpress.com/2011/06/03/name-change-of-wegners-granulomatosis/

[17] Hoffman G. WG or VF, what's in a name? History of the Vasculitis Foundation [Letter]. Vasculitis Foundation [website]. 2006 [cited 2012 Jul 20].

[18] ALS Association [website]. About ALS. 2004 Jul 29 [cited 2012 Jul 21] Available from: http://www.alsa.org/about-als/

[19] The Free Dictionary by Farlex [website]. Bipolar disorder. 2008 [cited 2012 Jul 21]. Available from: http://medical-dictionary.thefreedictionary.com/bipolar+disorder

[20] Hagan P. Manic depression has been rebranded as bipolar... But are so many of us really mentally ill? Daily Mail Online [website]. 2011 Apr 18 [cited 2017 Sep 1]. Available from: http:// www.dailymail.co.uk/health/article-1378299/Manic-depression-rebranded-bipolar--But-really-mentally-ill.html

[21] Today's Caregiver [website]. A brief history of bipolar disorder. 2002 Jan 31 [cited 2012 Jul 21]. Available from: http:// www.caregiver.com/channels/bipolar/articles/brief_history.htm

[22] Dainton T. Huntington's disease... What's in a name? Health Mad [website]. 2011 Feb 27 [cited 2012 Jul 21] Available from: http:// healthmad.com/conditions-and-diseases/huntingtons-disease-whats-in-a-name/

[23] Medicine Net [website]. Huntington's disease. c1996-2013 [cited 2012 Jul 21]. Available from: http://www.medicinenet.com/

huntington_disease/article.htm

[24] Wikipedia contributors. Huntington's disease. Wikipedia, The Free Encyclopedia [Internet]. 2013 Mar 26 [cited 2012 Jul 21]. Available from: http://en.wikipedia.org/wiki/Huntington's_disease

[25] Esserman LJ, Thompson IM, Reid B. Overdiagnosis and overtreatment in cancer: An opportunity for improvement. JAMA. 2013 Aug 28 [cited 2017 Jul 1];310(8):797-798. DOI:10.1001/jama. 2013.108415

[26] Parker-Pope T. Cancer definition needs to change, scientists say. The Age World [website]. 2013 Jul 30 [cited 2017 Jul 17]. Available from: http://www.theage.com.au/world/cancer-definition-needs-to-change-scientists-say-20130730-2qvrk.html

[27] Parker-Pope T. Cancer definition needs to change, scientists say. (See footnote Chapter 10.)

CHAPTER ELEVEN
ANSWERING ARGUMENTS AGAINST RD

Telling the truth about RD can only help patients and rheumatology.

Responses to 5 possible objections to the term "rheumatoid disease"

In the past few years, I have encountered little opposition to updating the term "rheumatoid arthritis" to "rheumatoid disease." However, in the hopes of advancing discussion about this change, I want to address possible objections to it. Some of them are opinions I myself once held, before I learned so much about RD.

OBJECTION ONE: "Patients don't get to decide these things; doctors do."

ANSWER ONE: The first thing to recognize is that the movement to update the name of RD is not exclusively a patient movement. The movement has included physicians, researchers, caregivers, and concerned people who are not rheumatoid patients themselves. Agreement that change is needed is a result of common experiences of encountering the failures and roadblocks generated by the use of the term "arthritis."

ANSWER TWO: Second, I would ask: Why not? *Why shouldn't patients have more of a voice than anyone else since they have the most at stake?*

The name change would likely spur more research—a direct benefit to patients. They would also gain from increased understanding and visibility of RD. Patients are in desperate need of awareness of the scope and seriousness of this disease for many reasons. Here are five:

- **Accommodations:** People with rheumatoid disease (PRD) need accommodations of disabilities so that they can be employed as long as possible. Accommodations are often more difficult to acquire because of the lack of awareness about the disease.

- **Assistance:** PRD often require physical assistance in work or social situations in order to participate in daily life events. Historically, the confusion about the nature of the disease has greatly hindered their ability to receive help.

- **Medical care:** Lack of awareness about the systemic nature of the disease results in inadequate treatment of the extra-articular aspects of the disease. PRD also receive fewer medical screening tests and less preventive care regardless of their increased risk of cancer and other comorbidities (see Chapter 9).[1]

- **Disability:** Disability claims of PRD are commonly rejected, partly as a result of confusion between rheumatoid disease and arthritis (osteoarthritis).

- **Research:** While an increase in research dollars would benefit investigators and the profession of rheumatology, patients would benefit most. The majority of people with this disease do not have effective treatments and continue to suffer progressive damage and shortened lifespan.

ANSWER THREE: There is already a consensus among patients to change the name. Thousands of PRD have already adopted the term, and the Rheumatoid Patient Foundation has endorsed the change. In the age of patient engagement and empowerment, people suffering with a life-altering and mortality-increasing disease refuse to wait any longer for someone else to take up their case and make the changes that will alter the course of their lives. In an age when most adults search for health information online,[2] it is no surprise that patients connect with one another to find a solution to this problem.

Chapters 12 and 13 explain more about what you can do to encourage this change.

OBJECTION TWO: What about the ICD (International Classification of Diseases) code?

ANSWER: Diagnostic codes have become a central part of the way healthcare professionals classify illnesses for the purpose of payment for medical treatment. Each illness is identified by a specific code. The ICD-9 code for "rheumatoid arthritis" was 714; and the ICD-10 codes are M05 and M06. Dozens of subclassifications exist, many of them illogical to one who is educated about the disease, such as "Rheumatoid arthritis with rheumatoid factor of left ankle and foot without organ or systems involvement."

While many argue that the use of diagnostic codes is a less-than-ideal method of computing delivered care, use of diagnostic codes will likely remain a part of healthcare systems for the foreseeable future. However, there is no reason changes cannot be managed and updated. The ICD is obviously amended as medical knowledge expands. New diagnoses are added and corrections are made as needed.

OBJECTION THREE: But what will happen to the nickname of the disease "RA"?

ANSWER: First, this is not a serious counter to the substantive arguments in this book. However, it is an objection that I have heard and I will address it here.

Second, rheumatoid arthritis is not the leading reference for the letters "RA." The most popular meaning of the term "RA" in American life is probably "Resident Assistant," a post in most dormitory buildings in thousands of colleges and universities across the country. Online and worldwide, the term "Ra" is the name of the Sun-god of ancient Egypt.

Actually, an easy way to demonstrate that "RA" is not the best way to denote rheumatoid disease is to search "RA" on Google. The most popular results often do not have anything to do with this disease.

Abbreviations and acronyms are often shared by the sheer virtue of the fact that there are only 26 letters in the English alphabet. Out of the thousands of examples that could be given, the following are adequate to make the point.

1. In recent years, arthritis has been called "osteoarthritis" or "OA." However "OA" has been used for almost 6 decades in the U.S. to signify Overeaters Anonymous, the top result on Google for "OA." That is the OA that more Americans grew up with and recognize. The other common use for OA is the Order of the Arrow, a one-hundred-year-old National Honor Society of the Boy Scouts of America. When millions of scouting families say

"OA," they do not mean arthritis. There are so many meanings for OA that Wikipedia has a disambiguation page dedicated to it.[3]

2. At least three common things share the acronym PSA: The most common is probably public service announcement, usually referred to as a "PSA." However, PsA is the abbreviation often used by rheumatologists for psoriatic arthritis, an inflammatory autoimmune disease. Probably the most common medical use of PSA in the U.S. is to signify a common cancer screening test recommended for men age 50 and older, the prostate-specific antigen.

3. The American College of Rheumatology regularly uses the acronym ACR. However, since 1923, the American College of Radiology has used "ACR" and it is their registered trademark.[4] Google search shows several pages of different results for the acronym ACR. It must be noted there have been several incarnations of the American College of Rheumatology, with restyled acronyms, including the American Committee for the Control of Rheumatism, the American Association for the Study and Control of Rheumatism, and the American Rheumatism Association. "In 1985, the ARA formally separated from the Arthritis Foundation, with which it had merged in 1965, and renamed itself the American College of Rheumatology (ACR)."[5] Surely, the ACR can acknowledge there sometimes exists a need for updating a name.

As stated above, loyalty to a nickname for a disease is not a serious rationale for retaining the term "arthritis" as the label to identify a disease. The process of change will take time to complete, and, if one prefers, the acronym RA/RD could be used alongside RD in the meantime. Many patients already do this.

OBJECTION FOUR: "Changing the name is a waste of time that could be spent on RA awareness."

ANSWER: It is never a waste of time to do what is right! Even if this were not the case, changing the name of RA is also the most expedient way to improve communication, reduce common misconceptions, and improve awareness of rheumatoid disease. *No other single action could do more to advance public understanding of what the victims of this disease endure than to call it by what it is: a disease.*

I hope that the one physician who made this objection publicly will change his mind after reading this book. Having worked as a volunteer several years, increasing RA awareness and providing resources for millions of people living with the disease, I've obviously invested my life in the goal of RA awareness. As explained in Chapter 1, I've become convinced that comprehensive "RA awareness" will not be accomplished without updating the terminology.

OBJECTION FIVE: Without "arthritis," there is no "rheumatoid."

ANSWER: Current diagnostic criteria do theoretically make it true that "RA does not exist without joint inflammation" (or to be precise, synovitis in small joints). However, this statement is also disproved by the existence of both *extra-articular disease* and a *pre-articular disease* discussed in this book. In the future, better tests will enable earlier identification of the presence of the disease and better measurement of disease without conspicuous joint swelling.

Rheumatoid disease is a systemic disease that can be active in a person's body unrecognized for a period of years before joint symptoms become evident. Initial symptoms may or may not be joint symptoms. When joint symptoms eventually become evident to the patient, there is often additional time before there are enough consistent, visible symptoms for a doctor to recognize "arthritis," literally "inflamed joints." Furthermore, a specific diagnosis of "rheumatoid arthritis" is not given until a doctor agrees that a patient has satisfied precise criteria for RA diagnosis, which usually means additional time. (See Chapter 2 for more on the extended time between initiation of symptoms and diagnosis.)

Most doctors only acknowledge the presence of RA/RD with obvious joint inflammation in a specific combination of joints. Now, research finally shows what patients have known for centuries: that the disease exists beyond visibly swollen fingers. If you are a health care professional or have concern for a person who is living with rheumatoid disease, I strongly urge you to become more informed about extra-articular dangers of the disease, both constitutional and organ-related.

On behalf of rheumatoid patients, I will continue to advocate for more thorough research as well as ways to identify and treat the disease at an earlier stage. I will also continue to inform patients about current research, the need for preventive care, and the importance of a comprehensive approach to disease treatment. Perhaps the most pivotal area in which I hope to bring change is to encourage health care providers to adopt a broader approach to rheumatoid disease.

Lives can be saved by simply recognizing that extra-articular disease is not rare and that rheumatoid disease exists beyond arthritis.

---

[1] Kremers et al. Preventive medical services among patients with

rheumatoid arthritis. (See footnote Chapter 9.)

[2] Fox S, Duggan M. Health online 2013. Pew Research Center [website]. 2013 Jan 15 [cited 2017 Mar 22]. Available from: http://www.pewinternet.org/2013/01/15/health-online-2013/

[3] Wikipedia contributors. OA. Wikipedia, The Free Encyclopedia [Internet]; 2017 Jan 10, 06:01 UTC [cited 2017 Mar 22]. Available from: https://en.wikipedia.org/w/index.php?title=OA&oldid=759274419.

[4] American College of Radiology [website]. Legal. 2004–2017 [cited 2017 Mar 22]. Available from: https://www.acr.org/Legal

[5] Antonelli MJ, Calabrese CM, Calabrese LH, Kushner I. A brief history of American rheumatology. The Rheumatologist [website]. 2015 Dec 16 [cited 2017 Mar 22]. Available from: http://www.the-rheumatologist.org/article/a-brief-history-of-american-rheumatology/

CHAPTER TWELVE
SIMPLE STEPS TO HELP MILLIONS OF PEOPLE

The simplest step to address the dangers of rheumatoid disease is to throw off the mask of "arthritis."

Learning to think of RD as a lung disease as much as a hand disease

Early in my life with RD, one woman was remarkably sympathetic to me. Since most people I knew were exceedingly dismissive of my RD, her response made a great impact. This lady seemed to grasp my invisible experience—difficulty walking, standing, cutting my food... And I learned why: her late husband had had the disease.

Over time, she shared with me his particular struggles and the ways he had adapted in order to do as much as possible. As his condition worsened, he needed a lot of help. I felt alone living in such severe pain and struggling to manage, so her accounts of his struggles were meaningful to me. Yet one thing about his story was puzzling: he also had a lung disease which concerned his doctors and friends much more than the RD. As if it were a secret, my friend whispered to me over and over that it was always the RD that was the heavier burden—despite what others thought. Nevertheless, the doctors claimed it was the lung disease that took his life.

As I listened to my friend tell her husband's story, I wondered silently about the connection between that man's death and his discounted RD. Since at the time there was no way to know whether there was a connection between the two conditions, I never brought up my suspicions. Today, as I review the sections on rheumatoid lung disease in Chapter 6 and lung evidence for pre-clinical RA in Chapter 4, I think differently. Investigators recognize that lung disease is a common characteristic of RD. Mayo Clinic found the risk of interstitial lung disease (ILD) to be 8.5 times as high in PRD as in those without RD. Looking back, it is unlikely that my friend's husband's lung disease was unrelated to his RD. It is probable that he died as a result of RD, and his doctors did not know it. The alarming facts about death certificates (see Chapter 3) make that seem even more likely.

Several years later and a world away, at a large medical meeting, I had a lunch conversation with a pulmonologist who was unaware of the strong connection between RD and airways —unaware that the some researchers have determined RD may begin in the respiratory system[1] (see Chapter 4) or that studies show airway exposures are related to RA risk,[2] as well as unaware that in 2009, the American College of Chest Physicians published recommendations for the management of pulmonary risk in PRD.[3] This doctor is not unusual. Medical books describe RA as a musculoskeletal disease; some mention the possibility of occasional "complications" or a slightly increased potential for so-called comorbidities, mainly in late stage disease. This is what most doctors are likely taught. Obviously, the consequences of such misinformation are grave, and steps should be taken to improve medical education related to RD.

Learning first hand that RA is really RD

While I could share hundreds of stories about those consequences, the foundation of this book is medical evidence for the dangers of RD, not experiences of patients with the disease. Yet, one recent experience has been so startling and illustrative of the hidden true nature of RD, I must share it. As I completed this book in 2017, it became evident the lung disease that my own mother has suffered from for over 15 years is in fact RD.

I began to suspect she had RD when all of her fingers suddenly drifted sharply to the ulnar side, a distinct rheumatoid abnormality. She also had mysterious joint problems, pain, and unexplainable "injuries" that made me wonder. Even with all the clues, I was still shocked when she finally told me she knew she had RD.

During the past couple of years, I have also experienced first-hand several of the issues I wrote about since I started this book in 2013. From reading research articles, I knew about several serious health threats related to my diagnosis. In addition, I had listened to desperate stories about them from other patients that I care about.

Still, it has been daunting to personally face these issues day by day—to see test results or the look of concern on my doctors' faces. I have also experienced many of the difficulties other patients have shared regarding diagnosis and treatment for these non-articular results of rheumatoid disease: loss of voice with immobilized vocal cords, skin vasculitis, heart rhythm irregularities, swollen liver, persistent shortness of breath, and other issues.

How we can fight RD

This chapter outlines specific steps that patients, medical professionals, investigators, caregivers, and policy makers should take right now. We do not have all of the solutions or cures to every danger of RD. However, there are several things that can be done now which will impact the health of PRD and change outcomes for future generations.

3 CHANGES PEOPLE WITH RHEUMATOID DISEASE NEED NOW

How can we change the status quo to help PRD be healthier, get better care, and live longer? These 3 changes must be made.

CHANGE ONE: Institute care guidelines that inform doctors and patients about the comprehensive nature of the disease, prompting PRD to obtain adequate medical attention for all aspects of the disease.

Clinicians who care for PRD must be made aware of screenings that ought to be performed, and what effects the disease is likely to have on a patient's health. Through their doctors, patients should also have access to accurate information about systemic disease effects, with special attention to serious aspects of RD that increase mortality. Patients should also be informed of all the joints that could be affected. Lack of adequate understanding of potential disease effects or common risks associated with the disease can have devastating consequences for PRD and their families.

The current notion of the disease as a "type of arthritis," emphasized by calling it "rheumatoid arthritis," has made this change unlikely. The name has become an obstacle to patients, doctors, and caregivers who hope to ensure adequate medical care. For example, it was the third doctor to examine Celia Veno who finally recognized the "floating knife" in her back as a result of her RD; and it was too late to save her life[4] (discussed in Chapter 6). Failing to recognize Celia's obvious symptoms of disease in her spine, her previous doctors had merely written prescriptions for pain medications.

Patients have often written to me or commented on my blog about similar difficulties obtaining adequate attention for medical issues related to RD especially when the patient has, in the doctor's opinion, "insignificant" arthritic problems. If a doctor is not aware of the extra-articular aspects of RD, he may not recognize a problem, or understand its significance. Doctors miss critical problems as they are mistakenly trained to focus on hands.

For example, in 1966 Conlon found cervical spine involvement to be so common that he proposed it should be used to help determine a rheumatoid diagnosis.[5] Indeed, as Carla Veno Jones learned after her mother's death in 2005, the cervical spine is almost always involved early in the disease course, and correlates with peripheral joint changes.[6, 7] Calleja says that spine joints have been found to be the most commonly involved joints in RA, after the MCPs. Even with the precedent of research, Celia Veno's first two doctors missed her RD spinal problems because they were trained to look at the hands rather than consider the spine.

Celia Veno was not a rare case. "RA activity in the cervical spine begins early, with 83% of patients in prospective studies developing anterior atlantoaxial subluxation within 2 years of disease onset. Activity in the cervical spine progresses clinically and radiologically in tandem with the peripheral-joint involvement. In fact, the severity of the peripheral erosive damage is strongly correlated with the degree of structural damage in the cervical spine."[8] And the sub-cervical spine is involved more often than is commonly expected.[9]

Recently, Korean investigators advocated early and frequent monitoring of the cervical spine: "Because subluxation could result in irreversible neural impairment, non-ambulation, respiratory dysfunction, and consequent death, its early diagnosis and treatment should be a priority in patients with RA."[10] Na et al. conclude their study with a recommendation of annual assessment of cervical spine instability in people with RA.

Yet, patients frequently encounter doctors who are unaware of these facts, having been taught that spine involvement is infrequent and rarely serious. Sadly, doctors often misinform patients that the spine is not involved in RD.

Tragic results of overlooking the seriousness of RD

Celia's daughter Carla is one of several women I know whose mothers died as a result of RD, during a time when doctors seldom recognized the impact of the disease on patients. Whether or not they themselves have the disease, loved ones of PRD are a unique fellowship determined to not see yet another generation suffer the way their loved ones did. I was always very thankful that my own mother did not suffer from RD herself, and I had written about that in an earlier draft of this book. But I was forced to edit this chapter as it became evident that my mom is also a victim of RD.

Either way, my mom has always been a member of our special group since her father was a victim of RD, dying at age 66 of a first-event heart attack, with no warning signs, as is commonly the case in RD (see Chapter 5). And her great-grandmother, a mother of five and my mother's namesake, died similarly at age 56, after years in a wheelchair from RD.

Several years ago, I listened to a talented research cardiologist give a speech explaining that he had never imagined that there was any need to study cardiovascular effects of RA before participating in his current project. He said until he was invited to perform his current study, he would not have realized any need of a PRD to be seen in his cardiology clinic. The fundamental facts about this disease must become routinely known for the benefit of the public: doctors, patients, and potential patients.

What patients and loved ones endure, whether it is death as a result of RD or a less serious situation, is a natural result of what is discussed in the previous chapters of this book: *RD causes several serious health problems much more frequently than is commonly recognized.* Cervical spine and cardiovascular involvement are examples of RD problems that are usually not acknowledged or treated. Other examples of RD dangers that are often overlooked:

- Laryngeal involvement that can cause airway problems is "often overlooked" by doctors because of focus on hand ("small") joints.[11]

- Morbidity and mortality of rheumatoid vasculitis are substantial with a five-year mortality rate of 30-50%. Although studies show incidence is 15% to 31%, physicians detect it in patients only 1% to 5% of the time.[12]

- Mayo Clinic researchers determined the lifetime risk of interstitial lung disease (ILD) in PRD to be 7.7% or eight and a half times higher than without RD. They estimate about one in ten PRD will be diagnosed with ILD, but acknowledge that their study may underestimate that risk.[13]

CHANGE TWO: Promote collection and presentation of data that accurately reflect the condition so that research may be conducted to improve recommendations and treatments for PRD.

Currently, there are numerous problems with the collecting or reporting of RD-related information. As discussed in previous chapters, information about RD presented in the media is often inaccurate. Health websites illogically blend information about RD and arthritis (OA), indiscriminately recommending methotrexate and gold injections or diet supplements for "arthritis" with no mention of "rheumatoid."[14, 15] One reason for this confusing practice is that media rely on sources that publish problematic material, including the U.S. government.[16] Consider the following problems with RD-related data:

- Frequently, RD data are mingled with data about osteoarthritis. Since the conditions are medically unrelated, require vastly differing treatment advice, and do not hold similar health risks, it would be more logical to list the data separately. However, the Centers for Disease Control and Prevention (CDC) frequently combines RA and OA data indiscriminately.[17, 18, 19] This has often resulted in meaningless data or inappropriate recommendations, such as suggesting a connection between "arthritis and diabetes" or using physical activity to "reduce symptoms."[20, 21, 22] Canadian Institutes of Health Research has similar problems, in one example blaming higher incidence of "arthritis" on obesity, although "the study participants were asked about arthritis in general."[23]

- Material created by the National Institutes of Health (NIH) to inform the public about diseases also fails to correctly manage information about RD. As the screenshot shows, a Medline Plus article on diseases having the symptom of fatigue, lists systemic lupus erythematosus, a disease quite similar to RD, but does not list RD.[24] Remarkably, "arthritis" is actually listed, a degenerative condition usually related to aging (or sometimes overuse of joints by athletes), for which fatigue is not a usual symptom. Strangely, "juvenile rheumatoid arthritis" (JRA) is listed as one of the diseases for which fatigue might be a symptom. Yet, its mention is parenthetical to "arthritis." This article is an example of the confusion perpetuated by careless use of the term "arthritis" to designate *either* arthritis (osteoarthritis) or rheumatoid arthritis (rheumatoid disease).

- RD-related data are incomplete because RD is seldom listed on medical history forms filled out by patients. Occasionally "arthritis" is listed, but without a distinction for "rheumatoid." Many PRD would not select "arthritis" on a form.

- Data surrounding mortality of PRD is known to be incomplete as a result of the extremely inaccurate recording of RD status on death certificates (discussed in Chapter 3) and inadequate understanding of extra-articular disease.

- Data from clinical trials with PRD are also affected by an inadequate understanding of extra-articular disease. People with known comorbidities are excluded from most trials although many so-called "comorbidities" *are actually rheumatoid disease manifestations*. Therefore, patients included in clinical trials may actually be those with less severe systemic disease.

- Many clinicians record patient data for scientific studies as a routine part of clinical practice. However, to the extent that a clinician is unaware of the likelihood of a particular disease manifestation (like shortness of breath), he may not identify or record it, making the data from questionnaires or other exams incomplete. Even so, when the data is later interpreted, researchers may assume it is complete, possibly leading to wrong conclusions. Several studies quoted in this book show that systemic RD manifestations are often missed unless specific tests are performed, such as an ultrasound of arteries to measure their thickness to look for CVD or a high-resolution CT scan to look for ILD.

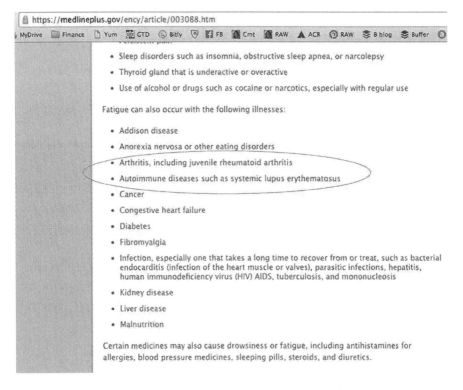

Careful scrutiny should be exercised when establishing rates of any RD manifestations.

As Fleming et al. recognized in 1976, clinician methods and expectations can be very powerful when investigating systemic disease manifestations. More accurate data would be obtained by systematically assessing consecutive patients with a comprehensive approach. They observed: "The high overall incidence of systemic manifestations that we found may be related to the comprehensive data we obtained by examining the patients systematically every four months. The incidence of symptoms overall was much greater than at any single visit. This suggests the intermittent nature of many of these disease features and shows the different disease picture seen with close monitoring, in contrast to that seen with isolated assessment of point prevalence."[25] Even though cardiovascular disease was not included, Fleming found a high early incidence of extra-articular disease with 41% of patients having four or more systemic disease manifestations and only 8% showing none at all.

In several instances in this book, I have pointed out the methods used in particular investigations. Some researchers have surveyed what has been reported in a group of existing medical records. Others have followed the records of a population of patients over a period of years. But, the most thorough investigations have involved using appropriately sensitive screening tests for particular extra-articular problems, such as HRCT for lungs or larynx. After selecting a group of patients, researchers screen every patient and sometimes also interview them to report symptom incidence as well. Obviously, this third approach is the most thorough and precise. *These differences in approach help account for the vast discrepancies in rates of incidence that are ultimately reported.*

The importance of accurate data for RD

More reliable statistical data about RD should be obtained and it should be presented accurately for several reasons, including the following:

- Clinicians and patients should have access to realistic estimations of risks for health problems related to RD.

- Drug developers and other researchers should be made aware of all disease manifestations, which could influence their investigation of the disease and potential treatment compounds.

- Accurate data about risks related to RD are needed for the public to have a realistic perception of the disease.

- More adequate research funding is likely to result from a more realistic conception of disease impact.

CHANGE THREE: Use accurate language to reasonably discuss RD.

In very simple terms, the most reasonable word for a disease is "disease." Failing to use that word can lead to illogical statements like the Mayo Clinic Blog title: "Rare Arthritis No Match for Woman Determined to Save Her Eyesight" when a woman's first RD symptom was eye inflammation.[26] Of course, it is impossible to have arthritis (joint inflammation) in an eye. And, the Mayo Clinic reporter obviously found it awkward enough to add the word "rare." But "rare" is not accurate since ocular involvement is commonly reported by patients and estimated by ophthalmologists to affect about one-fourth of people with RD.[27]

Making the simple change to use the word "disease" instead of "arthritis" would help patients more than any other change that could be immediately made. It conveys to them the need for medical attention, which could ultimately extend their health and lives. It conveys to their family the seriousness of their condition. It provides them with the best possible opportunity to get adequate care by communicating the reality that arthritis is only one symptom that they experience. Clearer communication promotes greater collaboration with patients in their care,[28] which is critical with a complex chronic disease.

As discussed in Chapter 10, names of many diseases have been changed to ones that are more suitable. Especially when more than one term has existed historically, updates are often necessary. Likewise, medical organizations want their mission to be clear and their names relevant and up to date. The CDC itself changed its name from *Communicable Disease Center* to the *Centers for Disease Control and Prevention*, a broader and more constructive name that better suits their current work.[29] And the American College of Rheumatology (ACR) has a history of name changes as well. It was once the *American Committee for the Control of Rheumatism* and the *American Rheumatism Association*. Then it unified with the Arthritis Foundation, functioning as the *American Rheumatism Association Section* of the Arthritis Foundation.[30] Its modern designation, ACR, is obviously more descriptive of its current role in representing rheumatology professionals and advancing the profession, especially through education.

None of these three changes—1) implementing guidelines for comprehensive care, 2) generating accurate data, or 3) using accurate language to discuss the disease—will be accomplished while rheumatoid disease is called rheumatoid arthritis.

"We must face the reality that anything with 'arthritis' as part of its name is likely to be relegated to a second tier of human suffering."[31]

The following essay is adapted from an article on rawarrior.com[32]

WHY RHEUMATOID DISEASE PATIENTS STILL FALL THROUGH THE CRACKS

The letter below is my response to the *Musculoskeletal Network* article "Cardiovascular Risk in RA Patients: Falling Between the Cracks?"[33] that reported on a new study published in *Arthritis Research & Therapy*, "Suboptimal cardiovascular risk factor identification and management in patients with rheumatoid arthritis: a cohort analysis."[34] University of Michigan researchers found that rheumatologists identify and manage cardiovascular risk factors less frequently than primary care doctors do and that even primary care doctors manage CV risk factors less frequently in rheumatoid patients than they do in the general population or in diabetes patients.

As you'll see below, this has been a known issue for at least a decade.

Musculoskeletal Network reported: "The authors speculate that many rheumatologists overlook cardiovascular issues in their RA patients, assuming (correctly or otherwise) that the PCP is taking care of that. But according to these findings RA patients do not benefit from the same vigilance for CVD risk factors in primary care that is offered for patients who have diabetes."

Letter to the editor of *Musculoskeletal Network, the Journal of Musculoskeletal Medicine*

Dear Editor:

Thank you for the February 8, 2013 article "Cardiovascular Risk in RA Patients: Falling Between the Cracks?" Falling through the cracks is a good way to describe a serious issue facing people living with rheumatoid disease: lack of attention with regard to cardiovascular disease (CVD) risk and other serious health threats that result from rheumatoid disease.

Studies have shown rheumatoid patients have a greater CVD risk than can be accounted for with the traditional risk factors mentioned in your article. Therefore, CVD risks tend to be underestimated in rheumatoid patients.[35] Most rheumatoid patients do not receive a cardiologic workup, despite recommendations of experts such as Sherine Gabriel (Mayo Clinic) and studies demonstrating the need for baseline or regular cardiovascular evaluation.[36] One study concluded: "Annual CV risk assessment using national guidelines is recommended for all patients with RA and should be considered for all patients with AS and PsA."[37]

Furthermore, rheumatoid patients often need to consult multiple specialists, such as ophthalmologists, pulmonologists, and cardiologists as well as physical therapists or surgeons to manage musculoskeletal issues related to the disease. This is in addition to the excessive level of "comorbidity" for various problems that require additional care from gastroenterologists, endocrinologists, or spine specialists, for example. Even so, preventive measures and coordination of care are rarely adequate.

I agree with the researchers' supposition that many rheumatologists assume primary care physicians manage these issues, while they usually do not. And, I suggest the following explanations may account for much of the discrepancy that these researchers recognize and that we see in our community:

> 1. Many assume that the risks are much lower than they are or that when these conditions occur, they are not

related to the underlying rheumatoid disease.

2. Rheumatologists may not be equipped to identify or treat the several possible systemic manifestations of the disease.

3. Years of living with inexplicable symptoms tend to make rheumatoid patients more hesitant to address additional medical problems.

Ten years ago *The Journal of Rheumatology* reported, "Patients with RA do not receive optimal health maintenance and preventive care services. Efforts should be made, on the part of all physicians who care for RA patients, to ensure that these effective preventive services are provided."[38] We implore the rheumatology community to work together with patients and with the Rheumatoid Patient Foundation to address this crucial issue through expanding medical education and public awareness relating to the systemic nature of rheumatoid disease and establishing of minimal comprehensive care standards.

Sincerely,
Kelly Young
President, Rheumatoid Patient Foundation

POSTBLOG:

While I appreciate the *Musculoskeletal Network* (MN) article, I have one further observation about their analysis of the Michigan study. MN wrote: "Rheumatologists may be well aware of the increased risk for cardiovascular disease (CVD) among patients with rheumatoid arthritis (RA), but a recent study suggests that they may be focusing on the rheumatic problem while passing the cardiovascular one to primary care providers (PCPs), who too often are failing to pick up the ball."

There is a clue here to solving this problem. As long as extra-articular disease is viewed as distinct from "the rheumatic problem," then rheumatoid patients will not receive adequate medical care. Non-articular aspects of the disease are not "complications" of rheumatoid disease. Statistics and educational resources must be updated to reflect the actual incidence of these issues in rheumatoid patients.

It's several years later, and I hope you will help me bring change

When I wrote that Letter to the Editor and follow up blog post in 2013, I knew that others considered it a radical position to suggest that non-articular aspects of the disease such as CVD should be considered as part of the disease, not "complications" of it. But, it shouldn't have seemed so extreme. As you have read in this book, there have been efforts in the past to broaden the understanding of the disease or drop the word "arthritis" from its name. Most doctors and patients have never even heard of those efforts. Yet it still surprises me how few are aware of the facts laid out in this book—facts documented in published research.

It's my goal to put this book into the hands of as many doctors and nurses as possible. At the same time, most patients and caregivers are eager to be informed about a disease that causes so many problems without clear explanations. Both groups—patients and those in the medical profession—will have to be involved in change. That is why I undertook the difficult task of writing a book for both of you.

I hope that you will become involved in creating this necessary change. I hope you will review this book at Amazon and other book websites to extend this conversation further. Loan your copy to a patient or physician who can do the same. Or use the special sales for multiple copies that will appear on Amazon or rawarrior.com to put copies of the book in the hands of those who can make a difference.

As for me, I plan to bring the book to the medical community in several ways, including giving talks at medical schools. Please contact me to help set up an event at your institution. I also plan to send at least one copy of *RA Unmasked* to Centers for Medicare and Medicaid Services (CMS) and the World Health Organization (WHO) (addresses in the next chapter). To get the phone number and email address of a regional contact for your country, go to this link: www.who.int/mediacentre/contacts/regions/en/. You can also engage them in conversation via their social media accounts such as facebook.com/who, twitter.com/who, or instagram.com/who. You can easily find social media accounts for the American College of Rheumatology and all of the other organizations and agencies listed using a search engine like Google.

FINAL THOUGHTS

In this chapter, I have shared some very personal stories of friends and family with RD. I have recounted my own process of revelation that rheumatoid *arthritis* is actually rheumatoid *disease*. It's true that RD has severely disabled me physically and prevents me from doing many things I love. It's also true that RD has frightened me as I've had to realize it may cut my life short, limiting the years I'll have with my children and grandchildren. Finally, it's true that I know and love many people with this disease. And because of what I have learned, I feel compelled to advocate passionately for their lives.

We now begin the process of recognizing the dangers of this disease and modernizing the term RA to RD, a term supported by evidence and history. The next chapter will outline steps you can take right now to help accomplish the change.

But let our final thoughts be directed to the people who live with the disease hour after hour, day after day, year after year. They deserve better—at the least they deserve appropriate medical care and encouraging social accommodations, yet many face frustration and stigma stemming from the term "arthritis."

Consider some ordinary examples of their experiences:

After a young mother struggles to make it back to her car from inside of a grocery store, strangers scold her for using a handicapped parking placard.

When a teenager explains to her friends why she is too sick to attend a birthday party, her friends whisper suspicions about her because they don't think she looks sick.

During a Super Bowl party, a commercial plays for an RA medication. The crowd agrees aloud that their friend who just got home from the hospital should try that medication so he can get back to life as usual.

A woman asks her primary care physician what kind of specialist she should see for her shortness of breath. He ignores her concern because he assumes that her many and varied health complaints may signal hypochondria.

A young twenty-something is newly diagnosed and expresses heartache over years of misjudging a family member with the disease.

A frightened mother emails me in the middle of the night after yet another trip to the emergency room with her young daughter with juvenile RD.

These are only a few of many thousands of experiences patients have shared.

Every day, people with RD are misjudged or have various tests or treatments neglected or refused because they only have a diagnosis of "arthritis." Patient stories are real to me because I have also had these discussions with medical personnel and insurance companies and family members who don't understand. And doctors or friends have rebuffed me because the description of my RD symptoms did not match their expectations.

The unfortunate language of "arthritis" needlessly adds to the suffering and loss of PRD. There is no good reason for that to endure.

Even if the historical and scientific evidence were not so clear, the impact on patients' lives is reason enough to stop calling the disease a "type of arthritis." For their sake, each of us can change the language we use right now to "RD." An effort by doctors to change the name failed in 1948. And even with a compelling beginning to a movement, another such effort failed in 1976. We can do this for patients now.

I'd give almost anything if the familiar lie were true—if it were true that RA just caused a little swelling in the hands and feet.[39] My eyes, veins, heart, liver, and blood would be fine. I wouldn't have trouble breathing, speaking, chewing, or walking... But it's not true.

Let's take care of people, take off the mask, and tell the truth—say "rheumatoid disease."

[1] Jancin B. Airways abnormalities may represent preclinical rheumatoid arthritis. (See footnote Chapter 4.)

[2] Hart JE, Källberg H, Laden F, Costenbader KH, Yanosky JD, Klareskog L, Alfredsson L, Karlson EW. Ambient air pollution exposures and risk of rheumatoid arthritis. Arthrit Care Res. 2013 Jul [cited 2013 Jul 5];65(7):1190–1196. Available from: http://onlinelibrary.wiley.com/doi/10.1002/acr.21975/full

[3] Kim et al. Rheumatoid arthritis-associated interstitial lung disease. (See footnote Chapter 6.)

[4] Jones C. Death by rheumatoid arthritis. (See footnote Chapter 2.)

[5] Conlon et al. Rheumatoid arthritis of the cervical spine. (See footnote Chapter 3.)

[6] Conlon et al. Rheumatoid arthritis of the cervical spine. (See footnote Chapter 3.)

[7] Calleja M. Rheumatoid arthritis spine imaging. Medscape [website]. 2015 Nov 14 [cited 2017 Mar 22]. Available from: http://emedicine.medscape.com/article/398955-overview

[8] Calleja M. Rheumatoid arthritis spine imaging. (See footnote Chapter 12.)

[9] Heywood AW, Meyers OL. Rheumatoid arthritis of the thoracic and lumbar spine. Bone & Joint Journal. 1986 May 1 [cited 2017 Mar 22]; 68-B(3):362-368. Available from: http://www.bjj.boneandjoint.org.uk/content/68-B/3/362.long

[10] Na M-K, Chun H-J, Bak K-H, Yi H-J, Ryu JI, Han M-H. Risk factors for the development and progression of atlantoaxial subluxation in surgically treated rheumatoid arthritis patients, considering the time interval between rheumatoid arthritis diagnosis and surgery. Journal of Korean Neurosurgical Society. 2016 [cited

2017 Jun 18];59(6):590-596. DOI:10.3340/jkns.2016.59.6.590

[11] Hamden et al. Laryngeal Involvement. (See footnote Chapter 5.)

[12] Bartels CM, Bridges AJ. Rheumatoid vasculitis. (See footnote Chapter 6.)

[13] Bongartz et al. Incidence and mortality of interstitial lung disease in rheumatoid arthritis. (See footnote Chapter 6.)

[14] University Health System for Bexar County and Beyond, San Antonio, TX. [website]. Treating arthritis. 2001 Feb 1 [cited 2013 Jun 28]. Available from: http://www.universityhealthsystem.com/treating-arthritis/

[15] Vann MR. 10 Daily habits for arthritis pain relief. Everyday Health [website]. 2014 Aug 22 [cited 2017 Feb 26]. Available from: http://www.everydayhealth.com/arthritis-pictures/daily-habits-for-arthritis-pain-relief-0216.aspx#01

[16] National Institute of Arthritis and Musculoskeletal and Skin Diseases [website]. Living with arthritis: Health information basics for you and your family. 2014 Jul [cited 2017 Feb 26]. NIH Publication No. 14-7050-E. Available from: https://www.niams.nih.gov/health_info/arthritis/

[17] Centers for Disease Control and Prevention [website]. Arthritis Data and Statistics. 2015 May 27 [cited 2017 Feb 26]. Available from: https://www.cdc.gov/arthritis/data_statistics/comorbidities.htm

[18] Barbour KE, Boring M, Helmick CG, Murphy LB, Qin J. Prevalence of severe joint pain among adults with doctor-diagnosed arthritis — United States, 2002–2014. MMWR Morb Mortal Wkly Rep. 2016 [cited 2017 Feb 26];65:1052–1056. DOI: http://dx.doi.org/10.15585/mmwr.mm6539a2

[19] Barbour KE, Helmick CG, Boring M, Brady TJ. Vital Signs:

Prevalence of doctor-diagnosed arthritis and arthritis-attributable activity limitation — United States, 2013–2015. MMWR Morb Mortal Wkly Rep. 2017 Mar 10 [cited 2017 Mar 18];66:246–253. DOI: http://dx.doi.org/10.15585/mmwr.mm6609e1

[20] Centers for Disease Control and Prevention [website]. Arthritis limits daily activities of 24 million US adults: Symptoms can be reduced with physical activity and educational program [Press release]; MMWR Morb Mortal Wkly Rep. 2017 Mar 7 [cited 2017 Mar 18]. Available from: https://www.cdc.gov/media/releases/2017/p0307-arthritis-climbing.html

[21] Chitnis D. CDC: Greater activity limitations accompany rising arthritis prevalence. Rheumatology News [website]. 2017 Mar 7 [cited 2017 Mar 18]. Available from: http://www.mdedge.com/rheumatologynews/article/132969/osteoarthritis/cdc-greater-activity-limitations-accompany-rising

[22] Rath L. More Americans report arthritis-related limitations than 15 years ago. Arthritis Foundation [website]. 2017 Mar 17 [cited 2017 Jun 24]. Available from: http://blog.arthritis.org/news/arthritis-disability-limitations-increase-cdc-report/

[23] Garrett N. Rising arthritis prevalence driven by obesity. Rheumatology News [website]. 2017 Mar 8 [cited 2017 Mar 18]. Available from: http://www.mdedge.com/rheumatologynews/article/132903/osteoarthritis/rising-arthritis-prevalence-driven-obesity

[24] Martin LJ. Fatigue. MedlinePlus [website]. 2015 Apr 30 [cited 2017 Feb 26]. Available from: https://medlineplus.gov/ency/article/003088.htm

[25] Fleming A, Dodman S, et al. Extra-articular features in early rheumatoid disease. (See footnote in Chapter 1.)

[26] Rivas R. Rare arthritis no match for woman determined to save her

eyesight. (See footnote Chapter 4.)

[27] Zoto A. Ocular involvement in patients with rheumatoid arthritis. (See footnote Chapter 4.)

[28] van Tuyl LHD, Boers M. Patient's global assessment. (See footnote in Introduction.)

[29] Centers for Disease Control and Prevention [website]. Historical perspectives history of CDC. 1996 [cited 2016 Dec 10]. Available from: http://www.cdc.gov/mmwr/preview/mmwrhtml/00042732.htm

[30] Pisetsky D. The ACR at 75: A diamond jubilee. Wiley-Blackwell, 218p. 2009 Oct [cited 2016 Dec 10]. Available from: http://www.wiley.com/WileyCDA/WileyTitle/productCd-0470523778.html

[31] Adams RF. An identity crisis for RA. (See footnote in Introduction.)

[32] Young K. 2013. Why rheumatoid disease patients still fall through the cracks. Rheumatoid Arthritis Warrior [website]. 2013 Feb 20 [cited 2013 Mar 30]. Available from: http://rawarrior.com/why-rheumatoid-disease-patients-still-fall-through-the-cracks/

[33] Musculoskeletal Network. Cardiovascular risk in RA patients. (See footnote Chapter 9.)

[34] Desai SS, Myles JM, Kaplan MJ. Suboptimal cardiovascular risk factor identification and management in patients with rheumatoid arthritis: A cohort analysis. Arthritis Res Ther. 2012 Dec 13 [cited 2013 Feb 20];14:R270. Available from: http://www.ncbi.nlm.nih.gov/pubmed/23237607

[35] Kaiser C. Cardio notes: Heart risk in RA miscalculated. MedPage Today [website]. 2012 May 29 [cited 2013 Feb 19]. Available from: http://www.medpagetoday.com/Cardiology/MyocardialInfarction/32959

[36] Mayo Clinic. Predicting cardiovascular disease risk for rheumatoid arthritis patients. (See footnote Chapter 8.)

[37] Peters et al. EULAR evidence-based recommendations for cardiovascular risk management. (See footnote Chapter 8.)

[38] Kremers et al. Preventive medical services among patients with rheumatoid arthritis. (See footnote Chapter 9.)

[39] Dooren JC. FDA panel recommends approval of Pfizer's tofacitinib. (See footnote Chapter 2.)

CHAPTER THIRTEEN
How You Can Help

After 70 years, let's make sure this change happens now.

If you or someone you care for suffers from rheumatoid disease, I hope reading this book has inspired you to help bring the disease out of the shadows. Maybe you are also saddened by the thought of children suffering either with incomprehensible pain or with parents who are suddenly unable to care for them or play with them. This chapter provides several ways you can help the cause of recognition of RD so that people can get the care that they need.

Removing the mask of arthritis is obviously a key to the recognition of the dangers of RD. That struggle began about 70 years ago, but it has been stifled by those who perpetuate misconceptions and insist the disease is "a type of arthritis." The facts in this book can finally help shatter those myths.

Our effort for change is exceptional because it is both a grassroots movement and one supported by academic research. This book is a big step, but what you do next is what matters most. Please take time to help insure that change happens now, so our children's generation does not suffer the same way.

GO REVIEW THIS BOOK!

This is the quickest way you can help spread the word about RD.

Go to RA Unmasked's eBook page to leave a review: http://bit.ly/RAunmasked

You can have an important impact by writing a review of RA Unmasked. If you've ever bought anything online—as most of us do—you know the value of reviews in guiding readers. Reviews also help electronic search tools to recognize that rheumatoid disease is a topic that people should know about, so they show the book to more viewers. If you write a review using the tips below, you are a vital part of this movement for change.

Some book review tips that might help you:

- Be authentic. Be yourself and say why you read the book.

- Be specific. Give an example of what you learned.

- Be creative. Add a little of your personal insights.

REVIEWING THIS BOOK ON AMAZON AND GOODREADS HELPS OTHERS FIND IT!

TIMELINE FOR QUICK REFERENCE

The recognition of Rheumatoid Disease

It has been a long journey to recognize that RD is a disease with systemic effects that cause harm and shorten the lifespan of patients. This timeline is a handy reference of some of the significant events in that journey. You can consult this timeline when you are explaining RD to someone or responding to an article online.

1812 – William Wells' classic article connecting rheumatism to a diseased heart

1898 – Aspirin developed by a Bayer chemist, being inspired to treat the pain of RD of his father

1948 – Bauer & Clark advance a model of a systemic approach to RD

1948 – Ellman & Ball advocate the use of the label "rheumatoid disease" saying "the term 'rheumatoid arthritis' is really misleading"

1949 – Bywaters' oft-quoted article on RA and the heart

1950 – Cortisone used as a remedy for RA – Hench wins Mayo Clinic's only Nobel Prize

1957 – American Rheumatism Association develops criteria for RA diagnosis to be used in research

1960 – Jonsson recognizes "the onset of articular symptoms does not mark the onset of the disease process"

1963 – Lebowitz bemoans the lack of attention to CV symptoms in Rheumatoid Disease

1966 – Conlon reports cervical spine involvement to be so common it should be used to help determine RA diagnosis

1976 – Fleming et al. prove systemic disease features occur early & are very common. 92% of PRD showed systemic disease within 4.5 years

1980 – Cervantes-Perez demonstrates pulmonary involvement in RA is distinctive and common, and that usual tests are inadequate

1987 – ACR updates RA diagnostic criteria, with emphasis on hand joints

2006 – Bhatia presents "Left Ventricular Systolic Dysfunction in Rheumatoid Disease: An Unrecognized Burden"

2007 – Mayo Clinic recommends comprehensive cardiovascular risk assessment for all newly diagnosed PRD

2009 – RAwarrior.com is founded

2009 – American College of Chest Physicians publish recommendations to manage pulmonary risk in people with RD

2010 – ACR publishes new RA diagnostic criteria, which emphasize "small joints" to include the possibility of feet for diagnosis

2011 – Rheumatoid Patient Foundation is founded

2012 – Several investigators publish studies of pre-clinical RA

2016 – Karolinska Institute demonstrates how antibodies associated with RA cause pain and damage apart from inflammation

2016 – Korean investigators recommend annual assessments of cervical spine instability in people with RA

2017 – Zhang et al. recommend all patients be screened upon diagnosis of RD to detect lung function changes at an early stage

2017 – Rheumatoid Arthritis Unmasked: 10 Dangers of Rheumatoid Disease is published

DON'T MISS ANYTHING!
GO SIGN UP FOR RA WARRIOR UPDATES
http://rawarrior.com/newsletter

WHAT PATIENTS AND CAREGIVERS CAN DO RIGHT NOW

1. Seek the best medical care possible. Seek treatment for any of the *10 Dangers of Rheumatoid Disease* listed in this book or any other extra-articular symptoms or

risks associated with RD.

2. Give a copy of *RA Unmasked* to a doctor.

3 Use the word "disease" to discuss the disease. There is no need to wait.

4. Recommend to friends and loved ones to seek treatment early for any symptoms that may indicate a diagnosis of RD.

5. Support the work of the patient organization that advocates for PRD, the Rheumatoid Patient Foundation: http://rheum4us.org

6. Sign the petition discussed below.

WHAT DOCTORS AND RESEARCHERS CAN DO RIGHT NOW

1. Seek to provide the most thorough care possible for all persons with RD whom you serve.

2. Use the word "disease" to discuss the disease with patients, colleagues, and in written articles.

3. Give a copy of *RA Unmasked* to a colleague.

4. Sign the petition below to establish Rheumatoid Awareness Day nationally.

5. Encourage colleagues to say "RD" and to join you in signing the petition below.

WHAT CAN EVERYONE DO RIGHT NOW?

1. Give the World Health Organization (WHO) your opinion about the name and classification of RA/RD. WHO is soliciting comments from the public regarding

disease classifications and definitions, scheduled to be updated in 2018. Go to this link online: http://www.who.int/classifications/icd/revision/icd11faq/en/

2. Sign the petition supporting a national proclamation for Rheumatoid Awareness Day: https://www.change.org/p/president-of-the-united-states-national-proclamation-for-rheumatoid-awareness-day

3. Send a letter like the one below to the agencies listed, addresses provided.

SAMPLE LETTER TO ACKNOWLEDGE RHEUMATOID DISEASE

Title: RHEUMATOID DISEASE IS A MORE ACCURATE LABEL FOR RHEUMATOID ARTHRITIS

To: U.S. Centers for Disease Control and Prevention (CDC), U.S. Food and Drug Administration (FDA), U.S. Centers for Medicare and Medicaid Services (CMS), U.S. Department of Health and Human Services (HHS), American College of Rheumatology (ACR), European League Against Rheumatism (EULAR), National Association of Nurse Practitioners, American Medical Association, American Academy of Family Physicians, American College of Physicians, American Thoracic Society (pulmonology), American College of Cardiology

Subject: Rheumatoid disease, a historical term that has been advocated since 1948, more accurately portrays of the reality of the disease commonly called rheumatoid arthritis.

Details:

We recognize that

- Rheumatoid disease is a systemic disease that increases

mortality through its affect on the cardiovascular system, airways and lungs, eyes, skin, and other organs;

- Joint inflammation is a significant symptom of the disease, but not the defining symptom since the disease does not begin in the musculoskeletal system;

- Common symptoms include fatigue, fever, stiffness, hoarseness, malaise, dry eyes, shortness of breath, inflamed skin or blood vessels, cachexia, and severe pain and sudden disability due to weakness in joints and supporting tissues;

- And, therefore that rheumatoid disease is not "a type of arthritis."

Research funding should be drastically increased so that per patient spending is on par with comparable diseases such as SLE and MS, and not limited to the classification of "arthritis."

Therefore, we seek to have the designation "rheumatoid disease" added to the ICD-11 entry for "rheumatoid arthritis."

And, we implore all whose responsibility it is to serve people living with rheumatoid disease (RD), commonly known as rheumatoid arthritis (RA), by providing them with adequate medical care, or by performing research leading to better treatments and a cure, or by educating or overseeing nurses, physicians, or medical technicians to do the following:

1. Utilize patient-reported outcome measures

2. Investigate symptoms reported by patients

3. Treat patients according to the most up-to-date guidelines

Finally, we implore all healthcare professionals to become

better informed about the systemic manifestations of RD, and work whenever possible to reduce the suffering and excess morbidity and mortality of persons living with rheumatoid disease. To learn more about the extra-articular effects of RD, please read the book *Rheumatoid Arthritis Unmasked.*

Addresses to write:

U.S. Centers for Disease Control and Prevention, 1600 Clifton Rd, Atlanta, GA 30333

U.S. Food and Drug Administration, 10903 New Hampshire Ave, Silver Spring, MD 20993-0002

U.S. Centers for Medicare and Medicaid Services, 7500 Security Boulevard, Baltimore, MD 21244

U.S. Department of Health and Human Services, 225 Tift Ave, Tifton, GA 31794

American College of Rheumatology, 2200 Lake Blvd, Atlanta, GA 30319

European League Against Rheumatism (EULAR), Seestrasse 240, CH 8802 Kilchberg (Zürich) Switzerland

American Thoracic Society, 25 Broadway, New York, NY 10004

American College of Cardiology, Heart House, 2400 N Street NW, Washington DC, 20037

National Association of Nurse Practitioners, Barton Oaks Plaza 2, Suite 450, 901 S MoPac Expy, Austin, TX 78746

American Medical Association, AMA Plaza, 330 N. Wabash Ave., Suite 39300, Chicago, IL 60611-5885

American Academy of Family Physicians, 11400 Tomahawk

Creek Parkway, Leawood, KS 66211-2680

American College of Physicians, 190 North Independence Mall West, Philadelphia, PA 19106-1572

DON'T MISS A THING!
SIGN UP NOW FOR RA WARRIOR UPDATES
http://rawarrior.com/newsletter

Glossary & Tips to Read This Book

Never let unfamiliar terminology intimidate you from reading about things that you need to know.

SIMPLE READING TIP

How to read sentences full of unfamiliar or scientific terms

This book was written for medical professionals and laypersons alike. If you are a patient, caregiver, or clinician, this book was written for you. If you find unfamiliar terms in this book, try this trick I learned from another patient-writer years ago: As you read a difficult quote, don't try to pronounce the unfamiliar terms. Just say "it" or something easy to yourself as you read it. It should be easier to get the general idea even if you don't know the word. Then if you want to, you can look up words you don't know, and then read the sentence over again.

KNOWING WHICH PROBLEMS ARE RHEUMATOID DISEASE

This handy reference list will help you make sense of the many ways rheumatoid disease can affect people. These terms are often misused or used interchangeably. There are some things that are hard to classify, but this chart will help you be more informed and sort out what you read—even beyond this book.

Rheumatoid disease is made up of 3 things

1. Constitutional symptoms – like fever or fatigue

2. Musculoskeletal disease – joints and connective tissues affected by the disease

3. Extra-articular disease – organs and body systems affected by the disease

Not part of the rheumatoid disease

1. Comorbidities – other illnesses and diagnoses

2. Side effects – problems caused by medications

3. Complications – problems caused by treatment, medical error, or random chance

GLOSSARY OF TERMS

acute coronary syndrome— decreased blood flow to part of the heart, usually caused by myocardial infarction (MI) or unstable angina

arthritis – "joint inflammation"

"as much a heart disease as a hand disease" – that rheumatoid disease should be considered a serious disease because it can affect vital organs, instead of the common perception of it as a type of arthritis

comorbidity – an additional diagnosis

complication – a problem that occurs during the course of a disease that is not an essential part of that disease

conspicuous swelling – obvious external swelling that can be noticed from across the room

clinical diagnosis – meeting specified requirements for diagnosis in the opinion of a medical professional

dyspnea/dyspnoea – shortness of breath

extra-articular – other than joints

methotrexate – a chemotherapy drug that impedes folic acid so as to interfere with cellular reproduction, used in the treatment of certain cancers and inflammatory diseases like rheumatoid disease

microbiome – collection of microorganisms within an environment such as the body

mortality gap – excess mortality in a particular group such as people of a certain gender or race

pre-clinical RA – rheumatoid disease that occurs before a clinical diagnosis, which might include extra-articular symptoms or joint symptoms that are not pronounced enough for clinical diagnosis

secondary condition – a less prominent aspect of an illness, as opposed to primary symptoms or comorbidities

vasculitis – blood vessel inflammation that can cause narrowing or weakening of blood vessels

ABBREVIATIONS IN THIS BOOK

ACPA – anti-citrullinated peptide antibodies

ACR – American College of Rheumatology

Anti-CCP – a common blood test for ACPA, anti-cyclic citrullinated peptide

BMI – body mass index, body mass divided by square of body height or kg/m2

CA joints – cricoarytenoid joints; small cartilage joints in the larynx

CT – computed tomography scan, also called a CAT scan, a type of computer-processed x-ray

CV – cardiovascular, relating to the heart and blood vessels

CVD – cardio-vascular disease

DIP – distal interphalangeal joints, the joints closest to the fingernails

DLCO – rate of diffusion of carbon monoxide from the lungs, a test of lung function

DMARD – disease modifying anti-rheumatic drug, prescribed in attempt to reduce disease activity in rheumatic diseases

ENT – referring to ear, nose, and throat

ESR – erythrocyte sedimentation rate

EULAR – European League Against Rheumatism

FA – fibrosing alveolitis

HMO – Health maintenance organization, a type of health-insurance plan in the U.S. that requires a referral to see medical specialists

ILD – interstitial lung disease

JRA – juvenile rheumatoid arthritis, also called juvenile idiopathic arthritis (JIA)

LV – left ventricular, referring to left ventricle of the heart

MI – myocardial infarction or heart attack, disrupts blood flow to a part of the heart

MCP joints – metacarpophalangeal joints situated between the metacarpal bones and the phalanges of the fingers

MS – multiple sclerosis, a chronic, typically progressive disease involving damage to the sheaths of nerve cells in the brain and spinal cord

MSUS – musculoskeletal ultrasound

MRI – magnetic resonance imaging test

NIH – U.S. National Institutes of Health

NSAID – non-steroidal anti-inflammatory drugs

RA – rheumatoid arthritis; a common term for rheumatoid disease popularized by the Arthritis Foundation in an attempt to bring all rheumatic diseases under the umbrella of "arthritis"

RD – rheumatoid disease; a term used historically and in some current medical literature to denote the condition popularly referred to as "RA" or rheumatoid arthritis. RD is used by many patients and some professionals as a more accurate term than RA.

RA-ILD – interstitial lung disease occurring in people with rheumatoid disease

RF – rheumatoid factor, an antibody present in about 75% of people with rheumatoid disease

RPF – Rheumatoid Patient Foundation, a U.S. non-profit formed in 2011 with a mission to improve the lives of PRD

RV – Rheumatoid vasculitis

PRD – persons with rheumatoid disease; as with PWD, commonly used to denote persons living with diabetes

SMR – standard mortality ratio, calculation of an increase or decrease in mortality with respect to the general population

SLE – systemic lupus erythematosus, a chronic autoimmune disease that can affect almost any organ system, including joints

About the Author

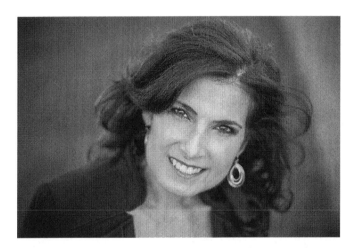

Mother

After earning a degree at George Mason University, Kelly worked at raising a family full time. At home, her ambitious DIY projects included landscaping, drywall repair, refinishing antiques, and spreading two tons of concrete stucco, as well as traditional home crafts like sewing, gardening, and canning. Every event or holiday was an adventure, from road trips to field trips to movie nights. She celebrated hospitality, and loved for every new friend to come visit. But her very best friends have been her kids. Her freezer was organized and full, unless she was cleaning it—which meant scraping huge bowls of "snow" for them to play with on a cool Florida day. Her five children, whom she joyfully homeschooled over the past two decades, have been the center of her life. Together, they filled the days with learning and recreation, spontaneous picnics, and days on the beach. Together, they made marshmallows, Winnie the Pooh crayons, Advent calendars, and dozens of sand castles. Her children were successful in athletics and earned academic scholarships. Most of them are grown, and they still make her proud every day. All of them, especially her youngest son "Roo," have been mentioned as she shares personal stories on her blog. *She calls this part of her life delightfully exhausting.*

Volunteer

Before RA, Kelly enjoyed volunteering in the community. She loved to make and send doughnuts, fuzzy pajamas, Valentines, and excessively decorated baby shower cookies. Kelly also worked as a volunteer teacher, writer, and editor for non-profits and churches, creating curriculum for children, teens, and adults, and delivering passionate messages on faith, church history, and Scripture to small and large groups. Her ministries extended to unwed mothers, parenting groups, and adult Bible studies.

Speaker and writer

Kelly has written stories, poems, and plays since she was seven years old. She learned to type with her kids using Mavis Beacon in 2002. In 2009, Kelly bought her first laptop and created RA Warrior.com, a unique comprehensive website of about 1000 pages of up-to-date information on RA presented in an engaging format. It is now the hub of a large, vibrant patient community. She has written articles for medical journals and magazines including *The British Medical Journal, Journal of Participatory Medicine,* and *The Rheumatologist.*

Kelly shares the RA patient journey through keynote speeches and consultations on topics related to healthcare, patient engagement and rheumatology. She has been an invited speaker at the American College of Rheumatology annual scientific meeting twice. She has helped to direct several grants, contributed to reviews of grants and CME, edited articles for medical professionals, contributed to social media leadership and coaching, evaluated scripts for health industry websites and programs for patients. She has partnered with government organizations and industry in ways that benefit patients by strengthening the patient voice and patient access to information.

Advocate

Kelly has received awards and national recognition for her work, but her keen determination is to ensure that future rheumatoid patients will not as those of the past and current generations. She has worked for over eight years to provide ways for patients to be better informed and have a greater voice in their healthcare. There are over 56,000 connections on her highly interactive Facebook Page. Daily, she shares compassion and hope with others, grateful for God's help to use her illness for good.

As a public advocate, Kelly brings not only an intimate knowledge of living with chronic rheumatoid disease and communicating with doctors and the health care system, but also the unique vantage point resulting from hundreds of thousands of interactions with patients. Through her writing, speaking, and use of social media, she has improved awareness of rheumatoid disease for both the public and medical community; created ways to empower RA patients to advocate for improved diagnosis and treatment; and brought recognition and visibility to the RA patient journey.

Kelly is the founder of the Rheumatoid Patient Foundation (RPF), the first non-profit in the U.S. that exists to improve the lives of rheumatoid patients. RPF has published research posters, videos, a white paper, posters, billboards, and several first-rate brochures for rheumatology offices. It has presented research at in the American College of Rheumatology Annual Scientific Meeting and participated in other national events to advocate for people living with rheumatoid disease.

Warrior

Kelly's life was abruptly changed in 2006 when decades of annoying episodic joint flares became full-blown rheumatoid disease, ending a very active lifestyle. She says the day before RA she could do fifty push-ups, and suddenly, she could not pick up her own purse. She had spent her life caring for others, but from that day on would need help to do certain things. The disease quickly spread, affecting every joint in her body, making it difficult or impossible to do many things she loves, including running on the beach.

Kelly lives every moment since that day with severe joint pain and has had frequent fevers, loss of voice, and shortness of breath. She fights every day to get as much of her life back as possible, being among the estimated thirty-four percent of people with rheumatoid disease who do not respond to currently available treatments. Kelly has spent at least six months each on several disease treatments, including participation in a clinical trial. For twelve years, Kelly has faced unrelenting disease, progressive loss of function, and medication side effects with resilience and optimism. She fights daily to maintain as much of her abilities and self-sufficiency as possible. She never gives up hope of remission or cure.

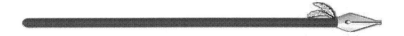

Made in the USA
Middletown, DE
21 August 2021